ELECTRICAL DYNAMICS OF THE DENDRITIC SPACE

The authors explain how the whole dendtritic arborization contributes to the generation of various output discharges and elucidate the mechanisms of the transfer function of all dendritic sites. Their alternative approach to conventional models introduces the notion of a functional dendritic space, and they have concentrated on a detailed spatial description of the electrical states at all dendritic sites when the dendrites operate. By analyzing the electrical dendritic space in which all the signals are processed, the authors provide tools to explore the spatial dimension of the transient events well known by electrophysiologists. They demonstrate the mechanisms by which the operating dendrites decide how, *in fine*, the distributed synaptic inputs generate various final output discharges. Their approach reveals the mechanisms by which individual dendritic geometry determines the sequence of action potentials that is the neuronal code. An accompanying NeuronViewer allows readers to monitor the simulation of operating dendritic arborization.

SERGEY M. KOROGOD is Professor and Head of Department of Experimental Physics at Dnipropetrovsk National University, and Head of Dnipropetrovsk Division, International Center for Molecular Physiology at the National Academy of Sciences of the Ukraine. He explores biophysical mechanisms relating cellular physical–chemical processes and geometry.

SUZANNE TYČ-DUMONT is Director of Research Emeritus at CNRS, Paris. She has been active since the early 1980s in the promotion of the notion of the dendritic shape as one of the most critical factors in the understanding of dendritic processing, and introduced computational tools for the quantification of the geometry of dendritic arborizations in her laboratory.

ELECTRICAL DYNAMICS OF THE DENDRITIC SPACE

SERGEY M. KOROGOD

SUZANNE TYČ-DUMONT

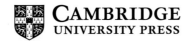

CAMBRIDGE
UNIVERSITY PRESS

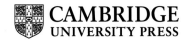

Shaftesbury Road, Cambridge CB2 8EA, United Kingdom

One Liberty Plaza, 20th Floor, New York, NY 10006, USA

477 Williamstown Road, Port Melbourne, VIC 3207, Australia

314–321, 3rd Floor, Plot 3, Splendor Forum, Jasola District Centre, New Delhi – 110025, India

103 Penang Road, #05–06/07, Visioncrest Commercial, Singapore 238467

Cambridge University Press is part of Cambridge University Press & Assessment,
a department of the University of Cambridge.

We share the University's mission to contribute to society through the pursuit of
education, learning and research at the highest international levels of excellence.

www.cambridge.org
Information on this title: www.cambridge.org/9780521896771

First published 2009

A catalogue record for this publication is available from the British Library

ISBN   978-0-521-89677-1   Hardback

Contents

Colour plate section is between pages 116–17.

Preface

Dear Reader,

We invite you to travel in space with us! This will be a very peculiar space: the dendritic space of neurons that is *the cosmos for neuroscientists*. It is mysterious and practically unexplored like the outer space we glimpse at in the sky. Curiously, we can further extend this analogy: the tools of astronomy can be turned from the sky to the microscope stage to explore shining brain stars, the neurons radiating their dendrites into the surrounding space. This was performed in the pioneering work by Paul Gogan and co-workers using a modified astronomical camera to image the microstructure of the dendritic membrane during the excitation of single live neurons in culture (see references in Chapter 14). The explorers of the dendritic space still have to invent the appropriate spacecrafts and technologies. As in cosmology, experimentation is limited, and mathematical and computer models are the only way of gaining insight into the nature of the dendritic space. The itinerary of our travel relies on these tools.

We start with a brief historical background to the dendritic problem and describe the origin of the structural data used for further morphometric and computer simulation studies of the dendritic arborizations (Chapters 1 and 2). Chapter 3 describes basic bioelectricity with emphasis on space. We show how charge carriers are separated in space and thus electric fields and currents are created across the neuronal membrane. An important generalization is that, despite multiplicity and diversity of channel types, the number of different types of current–voltage relations is restricted to three. Chapter 4 recapitulates the cable theory of the dendritic transfer properties with special focus on the terms of the cable equation which determine the electrical communication across the membrane and along the dendritic membrane. This issue is further developed in Chapters 5 and 6, specifying the voltage and current transfer along the dendrites. We highlight that the transfer maps provide an informative representation of the dendritic electrical structure. Chapters 7 and 8 explain how the electrical structures of an artificial dendritic path and of a branch bifurcation are built and how they indicate electrical relations in different dimensions of the dendritic space that are the proximal-to-distal and the path-to-path relations. Next the critical role of metrical asymmetry of the dendritic branches becomes obvious. Chapter 9 navigates in the dendritic space of biological neurons and introduces our library of reconstructed cells providing specific examples of metrical asymmetry of complex dendritic arborizations. Chapter 10 explores the electrical structures of single biological dendrites as the basic elements for constructing the whole arborization. Here electrical features related to elementary structural heterogeneities present in random combinations in the biological dendrites are noticeable. The electrical structures of the whole reconstructed dendritic arborizations of different types of neurons are analyzed and classified in Chapters 11 and 12. Relations of the electrical structures related to size, complexity and asymmetry of the arborizations are explored. Finally, Chapter 13 considers the consequences of morphological and electrical structures of the dendritic arborizations for the generation of output discharge patterns. These spatial–temporal patterns indicate some new emerging rules by which the dendrites govern the whole cell activity.

This book results from more than 15 years of cooperation between French and Ukrainian laboratories: the Unit of Cellular Neurocybernetics of the CNRS in Marseille and the Laboratory of Biophysics and Bioelectronics, Dnipropetrovsk National University and Dnipropetrovsk Division of the International Center for Molecular Physiology, National Academy of Sciences of the Ukraine. It originated in the form of seminars, lectures, published papers and notes for students. We have benefited from innumerable discussions with students and colleagues. To acknowledge all of them personally is impossible but we wish to thank first our collaborators who have co-authored our published articles and who were directly involved in various aspects of our work at different periods between 1993 and 2007. This book would have never happened without them.

In the French team, we are specially grateful to Dr. Cesira Batini and Dr. Ginette Bossavit. We should like to pay tribute to Paul Gogan who initiated the quantification of dendritic geometry. His vision was far in advance of the impact of computer science in biology. He had foreseen what could be done by introducing high computational technology in our neurobiological laboratory. His knowledge of electrophysiology, his wide scientific background and his generous participation in our work make him an essential person to thank. We would also like to thank the technicians, secretaries, programmers and photographers of our laboratories for their generous assistance and invaluable help.

In the Ukrainian team, Yuri Ivanov, Irina Kopysova and Vladimir Sarana valuably participated at earlier stages of our joint work on the dendritic processing. We especially acknowledge the contribution of Dr. Iryna Kulagina, who is the co-author of most of the results presented in this book, some of which have already been published, as well as unpublished data in Chapter 13. Her thorough and creative work provided novel dynamic electrical maps of the dendritic space which look sunny and bear clear landmarks of the determinative role of geometry in spatial–temporal electrical phenomena in the dendrites. We appreciate the creative contribution by Valery Kukushka who developed the NeuronViewer, a tool for interactively displaying spatial–temporal dendritic activity described in Chapter 13. NeuronViewer is available at Cambridge University Press site (URL . . .). Scientific cooperation between our teams was efficiently supported by the French Embassy in Ukraine and we are deeply grateful for that.

We want to thank our friends and colleagues Dr. Elska Jankowska, Dr. John Lagnado, Dr. Bob Liberman, Dr. Hans Lüscher and Dr. Gerta Vrbova for reading some parts of the manuscript and for their comments, criticisms and encouragement.

Finally and importantly, we regret that we can only provide an incomplete picture of dendritic spatial processing, but we are happy to open this space for younger generations of researchers.

1

Definition of the neuron

1.1 The biologist

The shapes of the dendritic arborization of vertebrate neurons is a unique property which differentiates the nervous tissue from all the other tissues of the organism. The neuron doctrine, which we owe to Santiago Ramón y Cajal (Ramón y Cajal, 1904, 1911), was established 50 years after the cellular theory proposed by Schwann in 1839. This long period of trial and error and of vigourous opposition by the adherents of the reticularism is simply explained by the great difficulty of recognizing a nerve cell on histological preparations (Figure 1.1).

It was only after the discovery of the Golgi method, which is a selective technique for visualizing nerve cells and their prolongations that Ramón y Cajal established the first fundamental concept of neuroscience:

All becomes clear in our minds. Why do dendritic arborizations exist, why are they so varied, so abundant, so extensive? We understand now. Simply to enable the cell to receive, and to transmit to its cylinder-axis, the greatest possible variety of signals, from as many different sources as possible; put simply, to make of the cell a microcosm whose connections to the interior and exterior worlds are as numerous and complex as possible.

He called the nervous tissue the most intricate structure known in the living world. He observed a great number of neurons stained with the Golgi method in a variety of species. The comparison of dendritic morphologies of neurons located in homologous regions of the brains of different animals led him to formulate what we call the *'shape hypothesis'*. It was in the darwinism context of the time and tuned with the comparative phylogenetic approach. During evolution, the structural complexity of the dendritic arborization is greatly increased and he also illustrated the idea that the ontogenetic history of a neuron replicates its phylogenetic history (Figure 1.2).

The evolutionary aspects of the shapes of cellular structures were also studied in the Moscow Brain Institute, where the concept that the higher we ascend the

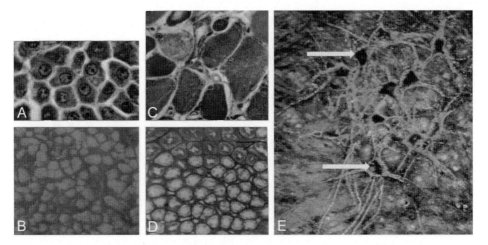

Figure 1.1 (Plate 1) The shape of all living cells of all tissues that make an organ are regular, similar and simply geometrically patterned. A: epithelial cells; B: tendon cells; C: muscular fibres; D: renal cells; E: the cellular bodies of the neurons are dark (arrows) with thick dendritic stems which divide into fine branches, the origin of which becomes soon unidentified.

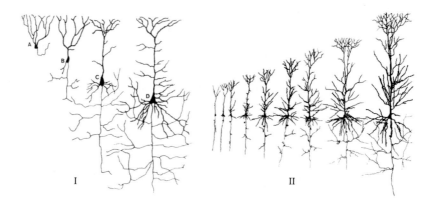

Figure 1.2 Dendrites of pyramidal cells observed in the course of phylogenesis (I) and ontogenesis (II). I: A: frog, B: green lizard, C: rat, D: human. The dendrites become increasingly important and complex. II: Growth of the the dendritic arborization of a pyramidal cell observed at different stages of development of the human embryo. (Adapted from Ramón y Cajal, 1911.)

phylogenetic ladder, the more complex become the dendritic and axonal structures of the neurons was developed by Sarkisov (1960). A definitive nervous system first appears unequivocally in the coelenterates (including hydroids, jellyfish, sea anemones and comb jellies) some 1500 million years ago. The nerve cell types evolve from unipolar to bipolar, multipolar and heteropolar types (Figure 1.3). The

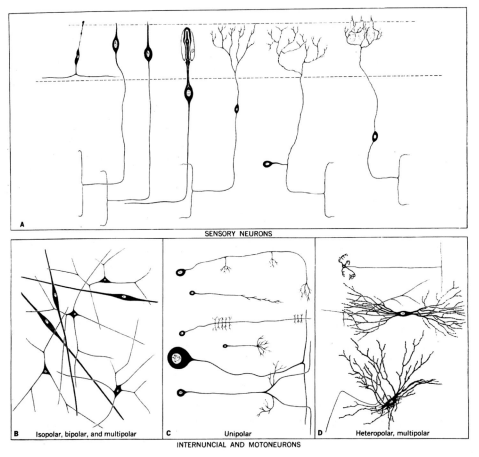

Figure 1.3 Types of neurons based on the number and differentiation of processes. A: Sensory neurons. The most primitive (left) send axons into a superficial plexus. In animals with central nervous systems the commonest type is a similar bipolar cell in the epithelium with short, simple or slightly elaborated (arthropod) distal process and an axon entering the central nervous system and generally bifurcating into ascending and descending branches. A presumably more derived form is that with a deep-lying cell body and long branching distal process with free nerve endings. In vertebrates such cells secondarily become unipolar and grouped into the dorsal root ganglia. B: Isopolar, bipolar and multipolar neurons in the nerve net of medusa. These may be either or both interneurons and motoneurons: differentiated dendrites cannot be recognized. C: Unipolar neurons representative of the dominant type in all higher invertebrates. Both interneurons and motoneurons have this form. The upper four are examples of interneurons and lower two of motoneurons. Dendrites may be elaborated but are not readily distinguished from branching axonal terminals. The number and exact disposition of these two forms of endings and of major branches and collaterals are highly variable. D: Heteropolar, multipolar neurons. These are the dominant types in the central nervous system of vertebrates. The upper two represent interneurons and the lower a motoneuron. (Adapted from Bullock and Horridge, 1965.)

excellent seminal book by Bullock and Horridge (1965) provides a review of early nervous systems.

The shape hypothesis is a concept within other principles operating in evolution. The evolution of progressively more complex functions has been made possible by the evolution of more complex structural patterns, hence more complex connectivity and greater differences between individual neurons. From lower to higher animals there is a scale of increasing complexity in connectivity patterns that is made possible by greater structural specificity and resolution in the morphogenetic mechanisms by which neurons become a highly complex system. How neurons grow into the fantastic patterns of connections that bring about their properties, which make in turn their richness of behaviours, remains unknown. We know that the driving forces of evolution have created the conditions for an enormous increase in the number of elements, in particular those in between receptors and motor neurons, the number and profusion of their branching processes together with the differentiation of shapes and connections. This structural complexity is the background that provides for complex manipulations of signals representing internal and external worlds.

An important contemporary concept of the neuron doctrine is that the neuron is made of several regions of different functional capacity facultatively interacting in complex ways, which will be discussed in later chapters. Some of the functionally diverse regions correspond to the anatomically distinct parts of the cell. The *axon* is a process specialized to distribute or conduct nerve impulses generally over great distances. It is smooth and only sends off branches at long intervals, if at all. It is commonly surrounded by a barrier of non-nervous cells called neuroglia inside the central nervous system and Schwann cells outside.

The *dendrites* are processes specialized for collecting information from other neurons, glial cells, circulating hormones and extracellular signals. Vertebrate dendrites are commonly highly branched, irregular in thickness, thorny and filled with cytoplasm more like that of the soma than that of the axon. No other cells can compete with neurons and their dendritic arborizations for sheer complexity of form and the extraordinary range of sizes that they display (Van der Loos, 1967) (Figure 1.4).

The *membrane*: all known organisms (excluding viruses) are composed of cells with membranous boundaries composed of lipid molecules. The membrane that surrounds every living cell is essentially such a lipid sheet formed into a bubble. The lipids are the primary component of cell membranes. Particularly abundant are the phospholipids, a class of lipids that consist of a sugar molecule (glycerol) linked to two fatty acids and to a polar alcohol molecule via a phosphodiester

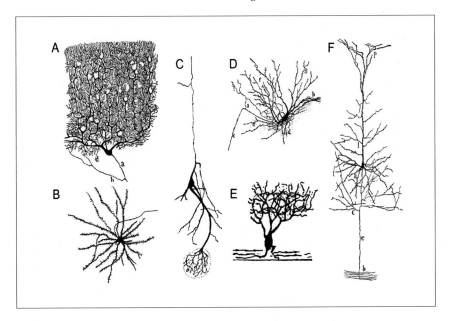

Figure 1.4 Drawings by Ramón y Cajal to illustrate the great diversity of the shapes of dendritic arborizations of the neurons. A: Purkinje cell (adult human); B: spiny neurons from the striatum; C: cell from the olfactive bulb (cat); D: motoneuron (cat foetus); E: ganglion cell fron the retina (adult chicken); F: pyramidal cell (adult mouse). (Adapted from Ramón y Cajal, 1911.)

bond. These molecules are amphiphilic, containing both polar and non-polar domains. Phospholipids form sheets by lining up with non-polar domains inward and polar domains outward. Channels are macromolecular pores lodged in the lipid bi-layer that make up the cell membrane and are positioned in a transmembrane orientation such that one end is in contact with the environment and the other end is located in the cellular interior. Integral membrane proteins consist of one or several transmembrane (TM) regions connected by extra-membrane segments. TM regions are 15–20 amino acids in length; just enough to span the lipid bilayer. They mediate the transport of ions and small molecules across the cell membrane along their chemical potential gradient. The other membrane components are carriers, which bind to a solute and move it across the membrane and protein pumps, which transport ion species against the chemical potential gradient expending energy in the process. Most channels in contemporary cells are highly selective to only one type of ion: Na, K, H, Ca, Mg or Cl. The selectivity is encoded in the amino acid sequence. The ligand-gated superfamily of channels is activated in response to specific interactions with small molecules.

1.1.1 Evolutionary history

Astrobiology, a new interdisciplinary field in science, explores the origin, evolution and distribution of life in the universe (see NASA's exobiology program: http://exobio.ucsd.edu/NSCORT.htm). Research is focused on tracing the pathways taken by the biogenic elements, leading from the origin of the universe through the major epochs in the evolution of living systems and their precursors. These epochs are: (1) the cosmic evolution of biogenic compounds, (2) prebiotic evolution, (3) the early evolution of life and (4) the evolution of advanced life. The principal goal of research in the area of the cosmic evolution of biogenic compounds is to determine the history of the biogenic elements (C, H, N, O, P, S) from their birth in stars to their incorporation into planetary bodies. The discussion deals with current evidence for the development of complexity, both chemical and structural, through the 4.5 billion years of Earth's history.

It is interesting to look at the recent results obtained by astrobiologists in this field and to learn about the emergence of membrane proteins, which are assumed to be essential for evolution from simple vesicles in the membrane to the simplest form of cellular life. Peptides are likely the first precursors of biopolymers (Pohorille *et al.*, 2005). The main thesis is that the emergence of simple ion channels is proto-biologically plausible. In fact, molecules capable of forming vesicles constitute a large fraction of organic material extracted from the Murchison meteorite (Deamer and Pashley, 1989), and were also obtained in laboratory simulations of interstellar or cometary material (Deamer *et al.*, 2002). The current discussion is how peptides have partitioned into membranes self-organized into functional structures and evolved towards increasing efficiency and specificity for adaptation and diversity. For example, the family of potassium channels exist in organisms from all three domains of life, eukarya, bacteria, archae, which speaks for their antiquity. Recently, structures of several K channels have been resolved from eukaryotes (Jiang *et al.*, 2003; Kuo *et al.*, 2003), revealing that the ion conduction pore and the mechanisms of selectivity are conserved within the family (Lu *et al.*, 2001). Analysis of the rapidly growing databases of sequences reveal that many eukaryotic channels have homologues in both bacteria and archea (Lu *et al.*, 2001). Many channels have been identified that resemble those in higher animal phyla (Hille, 2001). Given the enormity of time separating us from the actual events thousands of millions of years ago, only speculation is possible. Nevertheless, current opinion is that channels evolved from a common ancestor and that their evolution is extremely slow. The message that we shall keep in mind is that the main characteristic of the evolutionary history of channels is their remarkable conservation throughout phyla. The emergence of neuronal complexity relies not on channels, but on their organization and their distribution in more and more complex dendritic structures.

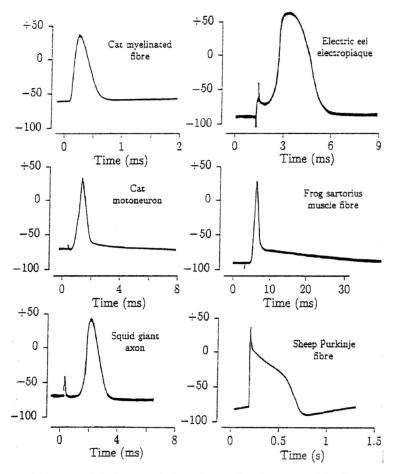

Figure 1.5 Intracellularly recorded resting and action potentials from several nerve cells: cat myelinated nerve fibre at 37 °C; cat motoneuron at 37 °C excited antidromically by stimulation of motor axon; squid giant axon at 16 °C; electric eel electroplaque at 27 °C; frog sartorius muscle at 22 °C; sheep Purkinje fiber at 32 °C. (Adapted from Bullock and Horridge, 1965.)

1.1.2 Neuronal excitability

Up to now, the properties common to all neurons can only be stated on the basis of a small sample studied electrophysiologically. All neurons so far examined are capable of an all-or-nothing brief electrical membrane change called the action potential propagating without decrement along the axons (Figure 1.5). As yet little can be said definitively about the evolutionary history of the signals used in nervous tissues except that the most characteristic of these signals, the action potential, is already present in the simplest nervous systems yet studied, those in jellyfish. Its common feature is universal without differences throughout phyla, although there are some slight variations in detail and mechanism.

To generate an action potential, the neuronal membrane uses some ionic channels. This operation is normally done by an intact neuron integrated in a live system, but it can also be performed by neurons extracted from their natural environment to be recorded in vitro and even by a small patch extracted from the neuronal membrane and sucked on the recording pipette (Safronov *et al.*, 1997; Wolff *et al.*, 1998; Safronov *et al.*, 1999). This observation indicates that the action potential is not only universal, but also the most primitive nervous signal.

1.2 The physicist

The neuron is a highly complex system. The concept of system is defined by a set of interacting elements, the structure of which gives its principle of organization. The term 'principle' indicates that the system is not fully described, but that data allow one to consider that the system is organized. The scale of observation determines the level of organization that is considered. A scale measured in tens of microns or even in millimetres deals with the macrostructure of the neuron, which is itself made of a microstructural organization explored by electron microscopy focusing on the smallest parts of the structure at a scale of tenths of micrometres or even less. The different spatial scales of the neuronal system span a range of three orders of magnitude. The crucial notion is that all these parts, from the smallest molecular to the largest cellular elements, are linked together to constitute an individual united whole. Any mechanical damage to a single part kills the whole as an operating unit.

Considered as an electrically distributed system, the neuron is defined by its active plasma membrane in which macromolecules, acting as intrinsic generators, are lodged. The macromolecular assemblies play the key role in the communication between intra- and extra-cellular spaces. Intrinsic generators are carriers of electric current which move the ion across the plasma membrane. Channels in the open state let ions passively cross the membrane along the concentration gradient. Ion pumps transfer the ions actively against their concentration. In such an electrically distributed system, the whole neuron is a functional structure made of linked elements. Any change occurring in a single element by the action of a current or a voltage produced by intrinsic generators is followed by an immediate characteristic change in the state of all the other elements. As in the structural notion of the united whole, we deal here with the same crucial notion of a functional unit made of electrically inseparable elements. Consequently every site of the neuronal space operates as a generator and a load at the same time. When the membrane generators produce unequal transmembrane potentials in different elements of the neuron, the voltage difference between the elements generates a current that flows between them. It is called the lateral current that is conducted through the extra- and intra-cellular space. The lateral current added to the currents flowing through the plasma membrane pictures the electrical space of the whole neuron. The main property of the neuron is to produce electrical signals which are funnelled into axonal and dendritic tubes. The shapes of these tubes determine the way the signals are distributed spatially within the neuron. Most important of all, the neuronal space provides the neuron with its specific electrical morphology and shapes the intracellular conductor through which all elements are connected.

1.3 The physicist and the biologist

Taking for granted that the action potentials and their instantaneous frequency at the output of the neuron is the neuronal code, this system of signals must be considered as the final product of a chain of stochastic events occurring continuously at the soma–dendritic membrane of the neuron. These transient discharges and their transmission through highly specialized synapses made electrophysiologists hover on the brink of major discoveries that Eccles (1957) made in the late 1950s. Intracellular recordings from mammalian spinal motoneurons and their synaptic potentials were a major breakthrough in neuroscience that came with new ideas opening the way for decades of intensive investigations. The drawback of such an important discovery is that it quickly establishes dogma acting as a barrier to progress. In his time Ramón y Cajal commented on this type of attitude:

That an idea may be mistaken or that a fact may be wrong matters little! The fact is simple, the idea is inspired, an illustrious scientist has put them forward; fashion, that indefinable something made up of idleness in judgement and deed, of respect for authority and total abdication of responsibility for oneself, takes over, influences other scientists by suggestion, and then, throughout their work, you see nothing but reflections of the trend they are following, nothing but proofs of the fact, confirmation of the idea.

Electrophysiologists have been fascinated by the recordings obtained with their tool – the intracellular or the patch electrode – and one of the dogmas in elec-trophysiology is to believe that the study of the transfer function between single or a few synaptic inputs and the output discharges is capable of explaining how a neuron operates. They forget that the output discharges constitute the space integral of all dendritic events occurring in the whole arborization and that they provide no information about how active dendritic sites contribute to the generation of these output discharges. Then the difficult question of finding out the mechanisms by which the complex processing performed by the interconnected active dendritic sites remains open.

If one assumes that the firing neuron is a functional unit that plays in time and space, one must admit that electrophysiology describes the phenomenon in time but not in space. Our hypothesis proposes to fill the gap between the temporal and spatial aspects of the same phenomenon by introducing the concept of dendritic space. We believe that the transfer function of the neuronal system, that is the functional link connecting a diversity of synaptic inputs with the adapted output discharges, will be further understood in terms of membrane mechanisms distributed in the dendritic space. As we know that the commonality in structural and functional design of membrane channels is antique and exist in all domains of life, it is only their organization in space, their distribution in the complex architecture of the dendritic arborization that can support neuron processing. We predict that the generation of all types of specific output discharges triggered by an immense variation of synaptic inputs can only be produced by an arborization in which a differential plastic contribution of all its dendritic parts is continuously selected by its electrical states.

References

Bullock, T. H. and Horridge, G. A. (eds.) (1965). *Structure and Function in the Nervous Systems of Invertebrates*, San Francisco and London: Freeman and Co.

Deamer, D. W., Dworkin, J. P., Sandford, S. A., Berstein, M. P. and Allamandola, L. J. (2002). The first cell membrane. *Astrobiology*, **2**:371–381.

Deamer, D. W. and Pashley, R. M. (1989). Amphiphilic components of the Murchison carbonaceous chondrite: surface properties and membrane formation. *Origins Life Evol. Biosphere.*, **19**:21–38.

Eccles, J. C. (1957). *The Physiology of Nerve Cells*. Baltimore: Johns Hopkins Press.

Hille, B. (ed.) (2001). *Ion Channels of Excitable Membranes*, Sunderland, Mass: Sinauer Ass.

Jiang, Y., Lee, A., Chen, J. *et al.* (2003). U-ray structure of a voltage-dependent K+ channel. *Nature*, **423**:33–41.

Kuo, A., Gulbis, J. M., Antcliff, J. F. *et al.* (2003). Crystal structure of the potassium channel in the closed state. *Science*, **300**:1922–1926.

Lu, Z., Klem, A. M. and Ramu, Y. (2001). Ion conduction pore is conserved among potassium channels. *Nature*, **413**:809–813.

Pohorille, A., Schweighofer, K. and Wilson, A. M. (2005). The origin and early evolution of membrane channels. *Astrobiology*, **5**:1–17.

Ramón y Cajal, S. (1904). *Textura del Sistema Nervioso del Hombre y de los Vertebrados*, Madrid: N. Moya.

Ramón y Cajal, S. (1911). *Histologie du Systéme Nerveux de l'Homme et des Vertébrés*, Paris: Maloine.

Safronov, B., Wolff, M. and Vogel, W. (1997). Functional distribution of three types of Na+ channel on soma and processes of dorsal horn neurones of rat spinal cord. *J. Physiol. (Lond.)*, **503**(2):371–385.

Safronov, B. V., Wolff, M. and Vogel, W. (1999). Axonal expression of sodium channels in rat spinal neurones during postnatal development. *J. Physiol. (Lond.)*, **514**(3):727–734.

Sarkisov, S. A. (1960). The functional interpretation of certain morphological structures of the cortex of the brain in the evolutionary aspect. In Tower, D. B. and Schadé, J. P. (eds.), *Structure and Function of the Cerebral Cortex. Proceedings of the Second International Meeting of Neurobiologists*, p. 81–87, Amsterdam: Elsevier.

Van der Loos, H. (1967). The history of the neuron. In Hyden, H. (ed.), *The Neuron*, p. 1–47, Amsterdam: Elsevier.

Wolff, M., Vogel, W. and Safronov, B. V. (1998). Uneven distribution of K+ channels in soma, axon and dendrites of rat spinal neurones: functional role of the soma in generation of action potentials. *J. Physiol. (Lond.)*, **509**(3):767–776.

2

3D geometry of dendritic arborizations

2.1 Brief historical background

The lack of methods of fixation and the lack of staining techniques seriously handicapped the earlier workers in their observations of nervous tissues during the nineteenth century. The story changed enormously during the last decades of the twentieth century when Golgi found that osmic dichromate fixation followed by silver impregnation gave pictures that could not be achieved by any other method. The enthusiastic description by Ramón y Cajal of the beauty of the successful Golgi preparations depicts for the first time the richness of these histological images:

Against a perfectly translucent yellow ground, you can make out, dotted with dark strands, smooth and thin or rough and thick, black bodies – triangular, star-shaped, shaped like spindles – looking like designs in Indian ink on transparent paper. There is nothing to interpret, nothing to do but watch and take note of this cell with its many moving branches covered in crystals, whose movements encompass a remarkably large area; this smooth even fibre which, originating in the cell, sets off from it to cover enormous distances . . .

The gifted hand of Ramón y Cajal produced the first seminal book on nervous systems proposing prophetic views on the functions of dendritic arborizations (Ramón y Cajal, 1911). But the lengthy and elaborate descriptions of Golgi preparations discouraged the students who were frustrated with this type of investigation and, influenced by the new results of local electrical stimulation, tended to devote themselves to the new promising approach of electrophysiology. The Spanish school declined, the last elaborate studies being made by Ramón y Cajal's pupil, Lorente de Nó (Lorente de Nó, 1922, 1934). The importance of understanding the nature of dendritic electrogenesis was stated by Lorente de Nó and Condouris who argued that all-or-nothing law could not be completely valid for the bodies and dendrites of neurons but instead suggested some kind of graded response action capable of spreading without leaving a refractory period and capable of summating (Lorente de Nó and Condouris, 1959).

13

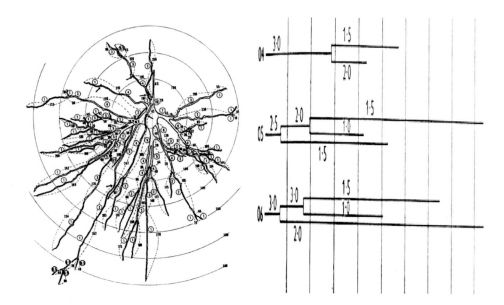

Figure 2.1 Left: An example of a reconstruction of a neuron of nucleus magnocellularis drawn from successive micrographs. The length and thickness of dendritic branches are indicated in the circle. Concentric circles are separated by 50 μm intervals traced from the soma. Arrows show sectioned and reconnected tips. Right: Method of graphical representation of the lengths of dendritic branches for a single neuron. 04, 05, 06 denote the first branches that arise from the soma. The length of the branches are drawn to scale and the branch points shown by vertical lines. Vertical lines are drawn across the diagram at distance equivalent to 20 μm. (Modified from Sholl, 1953, 1956.)

During the twentieth century histologists were looking at dead tissues and their observations remain qualitative. It is only in the two last decades of the twentieth century that we find the beginning of serious and continued quantitative studies of the geometry of single neurons. The Golgi technique stains the neuron in its entirety with the dendrites and axon and their branches complete. Only a proportion of the neurons present are stained but it enables very thick sections (up to 200 μm) to be cut; consequently the whole ramifications of the neuronal branching can be seen. Bok was a pioneer in the quantitative study of dendrites (Bok, 1936a, b). He attempted to relate the extent of the dendritic field to the depths of the neuron in the cortex. Later, Sholl proposed imagining that the soma is surrounded by a set of concentric spheres (Sholl, 1953, 1956). The number of branches intersecting each of the lines is counted easily and is equal to the number of dendrites cutting each of the imagery concentric spheres (Figure 2.1). He represented his results by a diagram (called later a dendrogram) showing the first branch of each dendrite.

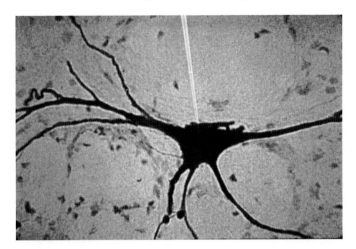

Figure 2.2 Photomontage of a motoneuron with a microelectrode implanted in the soma. Following an intracellular injection of HRP, all the dendritic processes are stained. (Photography Paul Gogan. CNRS-UPR 9041, Marseille.)

The length of the branches are drawn to scale and the branch points shown by short vertical lines. This was the first graphical representation of a dendrogram.

2.2 Single neuron labelling

The advent of new tools and new techniques enables neuronal geometry to be analyzed quantitatively. The invention of the microelectrode (Ling and Gerard, 1949), the discovery of dyes (Procion) for intracellular staining of individual live cells (Kravitz *et al.*, 1968) and the introduction of computers into research laboratories constituted a breakthrough in the quantitative analysis of the geometry of dendritic arborizations. An excellent survey of the state of the art at that time can be found in the book *Intracellular Staining in Neurobiology* by Kater and Nicholson (1973). A second major breakthrough came with the discovery of a new dye, horseradish peroxidase (HRP) providing the full potential of intracellular stain injections (Jankowska and Lindström, 1970; Czarkowska *et al.*, 1976; Jankowska *et al.*, 1976; Snow *et al.*, 1976). HRP soon became the preferred label because, unlike other fluorescent dyes, it resulted in a dense product without reacting to photobleaching. The HRP technique permits the entire dendritic and axonal domains of neurons to be viewed in great detail (Figure 2.2) and also observed at ultramicroscopic level.

The first reconstructions were aesthetically pleasing but their utility was severely limited by the lack of quantification. Data acquisition was first performed with a camera lucida (Schierwagen and Grantyn, 1986) and hand drawings or a tilt microscope stage (Mannen, 1966) or with eyepiece tracing and analogue plotter drawings. Satisfactory answers were not obtained until precise methods for accurately describing neuronal structures were developed. The practical difficulties involved in obtaining quantitative information have been thoroughly reviewed by Glaser and Van der Loos (1965) who were pioneers in implementing an online digital computer system for the semiautomatic analysis of neurons (Wann *et al.*, 1973). This basic principle has remained unchanged for the last decades although important progresses have been made in the technologies of the microscope-scanning stages, the metrology, the computers, the computer memory required for data acquisition and storage, and the implementation of dedicated softwares. A detailed overview of these technical approaches is described in a book by Capowski with exhaustive references (Capowski, 1989).

For any mathematical or graphical representation of the neuron, the two steps involved in the construction of a proposed neuronal model for investigating dendritic geometry are: (1) measurements of the labelled neuronal pieces and the acquisition of their 3D coordinates and (2) reconstruction, which must be performed after digitalization of the neuronal elements; it consists of a reassembly process reconnecting pieces scattered in the histological sections. Neither procedure is trivial.

2.2.1 Acquisition of 3D coordinates

The measurements of label pieces in serial histological sections relies on the quality of the optic of the microscope and on the precision of the mechanical system. As an example, the system acquisition built in our laboratory by Paul Gogan is described in Bras *et al.* (1987). A Leitz Orthoplan microscope equipped with a high-precision focusing mechanism (mechanical play $\ll 0.5$ µm), a ×100 Plan objective (oil immersion, NA $= 1.25$), an oil immersion condenser matching the numerical aperture (NA $= 1.25$) of the objective and ×10 oculars. For each point of interest, 3D coordinates are given by the position of the microscope stage (Maerzhauser EK 32), which is moved by three stepping motors allowing mechanical microsteps of 0.1 µm in X, Y and Z directions. Additional ×16 demultiplication is provided in the Z direction by the coupling between the Z stepping motor and the fine focussing mechanism of the microscope. The thickness of each section is checked before and after processing using methods described by Elias (Elias and Hyde, 1983). Other systems are described in Capowski (1989) and some are currently available commercially.

The measurements obtained by this first procedure constitute a database which is a numerical representation of the labelled neuron following a discretization process. The database can be used for vector graphic display, statistical analysis of the geometry or neuronal modelling.

2.2.2 Technical procedure for reconstruction

Once the labelled neuron has been digitalized, the neuron, which is a continuous geometrical object, is disintegrated into numerous pieces which are distributed in more or less distorted histological sections. The reconstruction process reconnecting pieces scattered in the sections requires a procedure of reassembling the disintegrated stained neuronal elements (Glaser and Van der Loos, 1965; Wann *et al.*, 1973; Zsuppán, 1984; Capowski, 1989) and is performed with dedicated software. It must provide tools for detecting suspicious data points, data duplicates and for merging the serial sections using manual or automatic optimization of section alignment (Bras *et al.*, 1987, 1993; Korogod *et al.*, 1994; Korogod, 1996; Horcholle-Bossavit *et al.*, 1997, 2000).

2.3 Dendritic quantification

Quantitative characterization of the branching pattern of an arborization is required for morphological description of neurons as well as for modelling their morphogenesis and electrogenesis. Quantification provides two types of parameters and characteristics: *topological* and *metrical*. Topological description deals with counting discrete elements of the branching structure, such as branches or segments, branch points and terminal tips. Metrical description deals with the parameters which are continuous and can be measured with a ruler, or a planimeter, for instance the thickness of a neurite, the branch length measured along its path in the 3D space, the distance in 3D (called *airway distance* or *radial distance*) between characteristic points, the planar angle between sister branches at their common origin (called *bifurcation angle* or *divergence angle*), and the spatial angle that envelopes a domain of 3D space containing a certain part of a cell.

2.3.1 Topological parameters

Quantitative description of branching structures is well developed in graph theory, a mathematical theory dealing with abstract objects composed of two sets of elements: a set of points called *vertexes* and a set of lines which connect the vertexes and are called *ribs*. A special type of graph in which the ribs (branches) do not form loops is called a *tree*. The graph tree is called *oriented* if a direction is defined on its branches. This abstract (mathematical) object is put in correspondence to a neuronal tree: the vertexes correspond to the tree origin, branch points and terminal tips and the ribs correspond to the dendritic or axonal segments connecting these points. Natural orientation of a neuronal tree is from the cell soma to the terminal tips. The trees are *topologically equivalent* or *homeomorphous* if they have equal numbers of identically connected vertexes and branches. Counting the discrete vertexes and branches allows the allocation of a number (integer). In an oriented graph, 0 stands for the tree origin (root), the branch emerging from this point gets number 1 and the same number 1 is attributed to the end-point of the branch. If other branches emerge from this point, they get sequential numbers, e.g. 2 and 3, and the same numbers are attributed to their end-points. Mathematically, any graph composed of N branches can be represented by a so-called *incidence matrix* (or *connectivity matrix*) of size $(N + 1) \times (N + 1)$, which is a table formed of columns, which correspond to vertexes and are indexed $i = 0..N$, and lines, which correspond to branches indexed $j = 1..N$. For an oriented graph, an element (i, j) of its incidence matrix is equal to 1 if the branch j is connected (incident) to the vertex i and directed to this vertex; -1 if the branch j is connected to the vertex i and directed from this vertex and 0 if the branch j is not connected to vertex i. The incidence matrix determines exhaustively the graph tree and allows the arbitrary numbering of the branches and vertexes, though it is more convenient to attribute sequential integer numbers to the branches on the paths directed from the soma to the tips.

In terms of graph theory, the topological elements of a neuronal tree are named. The three types of vertexes are the *root*, the *branch point* and the *terminal tips*. The two types of elements connecting the vertexes are *intermediate segments* and *terminal segments*.

The *root* is the point of origin of the tree, located conventionally at the soma. The *branch point* is the vertex into which one segment enters and two or more segments exit. It is said that, at the branch point, the parent segment gives rise to two or more daughter segments. Such a branch point is called a *bifurcation* or *multifurcation* point. If all branch points of a tree are bifurcations then the tree is *binary*. A part of the tree composed of a certain subset of connected branches and vertexes is called the *subtree*.

Several specific terms were introduced to label segments according to the number of terminal tips ahead, or to their topological remoteness from the root (Van Pelt and Verwer, 1986; Van Pelt et al., 1992; Van Pelt and Schierwagen, 1994; Van Pelt et al., 1997; Van Pelt and Uylings, 1999; Uylings and van Pelt, 2002; Van Ooyen et al., 2002; Van Pelt, 2002; Van Pelt and Schierwagen, 2004). The *degree* of a segment is the number of tips in its peripheral subtree with the pertinent segment as rooted segment. The *centrifugal order* of a segment is counted by the number of branch points passed on the path leading from the root to this segment. For instance, the segment originating directly from the root has the centrifugal order 0. The daughters emerging from the end of this segment have the centrifugal order 1 (one branch point has to be passed in order to reach these segments).

Topological asymmetry

The comparison of the topology of different trees reveals symmetry or asymmetry, depending on whether the subtrees born at each branch point are topologically equivalent or not. In case of most common binary trees, the *topological asymmetry* is quantitatively characterized by the *partition asymmetry index* A_p and *tree asymmetry index* A_t. The partition asymmetry index describes the topological difference between two subtrees emerging from a common origin and hence is *local* or *'within-tree'* variable (Van Pelt, 2002). It indicates deviation from an equal division (partition) of a tree into subtrees. The topological size of binary trees can be expressed by the number of its terminal tips (segments) n, by the total number of its segments $(2n - 1)$ or by the number of its bifurcation points $(n - 1)$. Any of these tree elements can be used to characterize the difference between subtrees (*the dispersion measure* according to Van Pelt *et al.* (1992)). If the two subtrees have degrees r and s, respectively, then the sum of these values $m = r + s$ is the *degree of the partition* of the tree into subtrees at the given common origin. Hence, at each branch point, a pair of discrete values is determined, (r, s) or equivalent $(r, m - r)$ assuming that $r <= s$ and $m = r + s > 2$. The partition asymmetry index A_p is defined as

$$A_p = \frac{|r - s|}{r + s - 2} \tag{2.1}$$

with r and s indicating the number of terminal tips and indicates the relative difference in the number of branch points $(r - 1)$ and $(s - 1)$ between the subtrees. By definition $A_p(1, 1) = 0$. For the symmetric partition with equal subtrees $r = s = m/2$, the partition asymmetry index is the lowest, $A_p(m/2, m/2) = 0$ and for the most asymmetrical partition $(1, m - 1)$ is the greatest: $A_p(1, m - 1) = 1$. The *tree asymmetry index* A_t is a global (*'whole-tree'* according to Uylings and van Pelt (2002)) topological variable, which characterizes the binary tree as the mean value of all its A'_ps, ranged from $j = 1$ to $j = n_p$ (n_p is the number of terminal tips or segments) or to $j = n - 1$ (n is the number of branch points):

$$A_t = \frac{1}{n_p} \sum A_p(r_j, s_j) = \frac{1}{n - 1} \sum A_p(r_j, s_j) \tag{2.2}$$

This indicator does not allow one to distinguish all the tree types of the same degree. For instance, for Uylings and van Pelt (2002), there are 127 912 topologically different tree types of the same degree $n = 19$ whereas there are 36 904 different values of the tree asymmetry index A_t, which is considerably smaller. However, other measures have even less discriminative power (see Van Pelt *et al.*, 1992; Verwer *et al.*, 1992; Van Pelt and Uylings, 1999). This description can be extended by adding other topological parameters, e.g. *vertex ratio* and *terminal/link ratio* by

Sadler and Berry (1983, 1988) or a similar measure called *1 minus terminal/link ratio* by Smit *et al.* (1972).

2.3.2 Metrical parameters

2D representation of trees

The complex 3D structure of the dendritic arborization is greatly facilitated when 3D curvilinear segments are represented by its dendrogram (see above Scholl's representation). Hence, the path representation of the 3D tree is formed by a system of parallel lines of varying thickness. Metrical parameters which characterize the extent and thickness of the dendritic segments in both 3D and 2D-path representations are the *segment length*, the *diameter* and the *membrane area*. The lengths of individual segments allow the construction of the 'whole-cell' metrical variables used in morphometrical studies and in simulations of electrical and electrodiffusive properties of neurons. Such variables are the *total dendritic length*, which is the sum of lengths of all segments constituting the dendritic arborization and the *path length*, which is the sum of lengths of the consecutive segments forming the path between a given origin and a terminal point, e.g. between the root and a certain terminal tip.

Trees in 3D space

Dendritic trees occupy a 3D space within the brain in a specific manner. Some quantitative descriptors characterize the extent of the tree structure, whereas others specify the orientation of the elements. An example of a relevant metrical parameter is the *bifurcation angle*. Another example is the *airway distance* or *radial distance*, which equals the length of a straight line directly connecting the origin and terminal point of the generally curvilinear segment or path. Naturally, the radial distance is less than or equal to the path distance between the same points of the tree.

The problem of metrical asymmetry

When trees are equivalent in their topology but clearly distinct in metrical sizes (e.g. in length or thickness), undoubtedly the topological quantitative characterization of trees is not complete. For example, unequally long segments may form unequally or equally long multisegment paths. Moreover, the metrical description is further complicated by differences in diameters which exist even between equally long segments. Although metrical differences between subtrees happen as often as differences in topology, quantitative indicators of metrical symmetry/asymmetry are far less elaborate than those used in topology studies. The need for some complementary description of metrical properties has not yet been met. Several measures can be proposed to indicate metrical asymmetry due to difference in length of sister branches.

Consider two dendrites of equal homogeneous diameter and unequal lengths, l and $l' > l$, emerging from a common origin, e.g. soma or a branch point. Obviously, this branching is symmetrical topologically but asymmetrical metrically. One natural quantitative measure of such asymmetry (dissimilarity) is the difference in length measured in physical units which we call the *metrical asymmetry proper*:

$$l' - l = \Delta l > 0 \tag{2.3}$$

Another way to describe the asymmetry of the branches is the ratio of shorter to longer branch lengths (measured in relative units) and this we call the *metrical asymmetry ratio*:

$$0 < k = l/l' < 1 \tag{2.4}$$

or the inverse value, which we call the *metrical asymmetry factor*:

$$\kappa = l'/l > 1 \tag{2.5}$$

One more measure is the *relative elongation*, defined as a proportion of the shorter branch length l that makes the absolute difference $\Delta l = l' - l$ in length compared to the longer branch:

$$\varepsilon = \Delta l/l \tag{2.6}$$

As follows from the definitions (2.3–2.6), the relative elongation ε is simply related to the metrical asymmetry ratio k and factor κ:

$$\varepsilon = \kappa - 1 = (1 - k)/k \tag{2.7}$$

Hence, for a given shorter branch length l, the length of the longer sister branch l' can be determined using the inter-related indicators of metrical asymmetry:

$$l' = l + \Delta l = l \cdot \kappa = l \cdot (1 + \varepsilon) = l/k \tag{2.8}$$

2.3.3 Complexity function

The complexity of dendrites is due to the presence of multiple branching points and hence multiple branches and paths. To characterize this property, one has to deal with discrete topological elements (branches, branch points, end-points) and metrical parameters (e.g. path distance from soma) indicating the spatial location of these elements, which can be described by a discrete function of continuous metrical argument. This is the *complexity function*. It is defined as the number of dendritic paths at various path distances from the soma for any dendritic domain. At zero path distance, the complexity function equals the number of primary dendrites emerging from the soma $P(0) = N$ ($P(0) = 1$ for an individual dendrite). As the path distance increases, the number of paths increases by one, when a bifurcation occurs, or decreases by one when a path ends. Hence the complexity function increases in the spatial domain where branchings prevail over terminations and decreases where terminals prevail. A reconstructed dendritic arborization is usually sampled at a discrete number of sites and hence the path distance can be measured discretely. In this case, the complexity function can by estimated from the histogram of path distance distribution of the number of dendritic paths. This estimate is accurate, as the finite number of branch points and ends which are definitive for the complexity function allows their complete sampling, unlike the practically infinite number of intermediate points along the branches. Demonstration of the use of the complexity function is shown in Chapter 11.

2.4 Data quality and morphological noise

Whatever the acquisition system and the data processing, it is not possible to exactly retrieve the real original neuronal structure because of histological, optical and operator-linked distortions. Since the development of a combined object-relational database (Shepherd *et al.*, 1998) which focused on different types of membrane properties to be included in canonical forms of neurons, new databases have appeared in the domain of brain-structure relationships (Kötter, 2001). As recently stressed by Shepherd: 'Archiving neuronal properties and making them web-accessible to integrating and search tools is a fundamental problem which is how to control for the quality of the data; many feel that this is the main problem to be solved before any widely accessible databases should be built' (Shepherd *et al.*, 1998). So far, there are no attempts to provide an estimation of the morphological noise which alters the geometry of reconstructed neurons. Published material and available databases do not provide sufficient information to evaluate this noise since only the final result of the neuron reconstruction is given and complete raw data are generally not accessible.

Our contribution to this important problem was published in 2000 and 2002 proposing a detailed method for checking data quality (Horcholle-Bossavit *et al.*, 2000; Kaspirzhny *et al.*, 2002). We suggest several simple methods to detect and evaluate morphological noise and its possible functional consequences in neuronal simulation (Horcholle-Bossavit *et al.*, 2000; Kaspirzhny *et al.*, 2002). We demonstrate that the two procedures (acquisition and assembly) involved in the reconstruction process introduce a morphological noise in any representation of the digitized neuron. Any neuron reconstructed on the basis of metrical and topological parameters is blurred by some morphological noise.

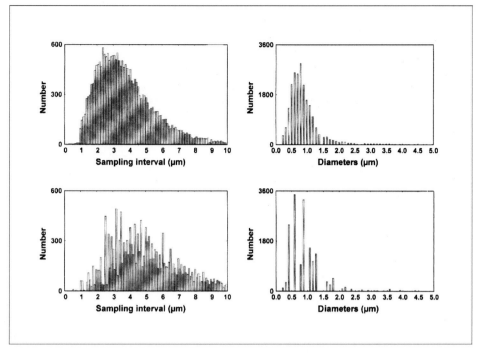

Figure 2.3 An example of analysis of sampling intervals and diameter measurements in two versions A and B of a frog motoneuron. For the 3D sampling interval (left), the distributions are built using a bin width of 0.1 μm and clipped to values less than or equal to 10 μm. For diameters (right), the distributions are built using a bin width of 0.05 μm and clipped to values less than or equal to 5 μm. (From Kaspirzhny *et al.*, 2002.)

Two series of stochastic parameters must be considered as the morphological noise. *The first series* concerns the digitizing process and depends on the combination of instrumental noise and operator skill. It is described by the accuracy in the measurements of diameters, X, Y, Z distances and topological coding. The quality of the morphological description depends on the sampling interval used to describe the changes in direction, the length and the diameter of the neuronal pieces. The smaller and constant the sampling intervals, the better the description of the length of the neuritic paths (Figure 2.3).

The second series of parameters is related to the reconstruction procedure for merging the serial sections to reconstitute the arborization. It contains the distortions due to histological treatments of the serial sections and possible topological errors. This evaluation can only be performed if the data describing the original digitized pieces (i.e. before merging and without corrections for shrinkage and/or wrinkling) are available. Number of dendritic roots, size and complexity of the dendritic arborization are sources of difficulties for matching the original pairs of

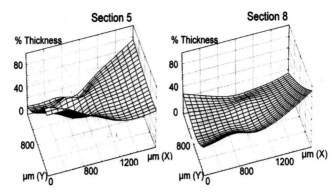

Figure 2.4 One example of analysis of thicknesses distortion in two histological sections of a frog lumbar motoneuron. The actual thicknesses observed after digitizing successive histological sections (examples of section 5 and 8) cut from the frog motoneuron are compared. Section thickness is expressed as a percentage of the original thickness at the microtome (80 μm) and plotted (B-spline area fitting) as a function of *XY* coordinates in the sectioning plane. (From Kaspirzhny *et al.*, 2002.)

contiguous points, now found in pairs of adjacent sections. Ideally, all pairs of points should have identical 3D coordinates. However, they are actually separated by random distances as, for light microscopical observations, the tissue block is cut into thin slices with more or less irregular surfaces. Furthermore, whatever the fixation procedure and histological treatment, they are unhomogeneously distorted (Figure 2.4).

It is very difficult to correct the distortions resulting from tissue shrinking and/or wrinkling. Although some computer algorithms such as the 'volleyball net algorithm' have been proposed to deal with such distortions (for review, see Capowski, 1989), the use of such algorithms may introduce even more distortions in the data since the physical model underlying the distortions depends on many parameters and is generally unknown. For example, it was shown that neurons stained with HRP did not shrink with the slices and that instead the dendritic and axonal arbors bent and curled due to the compression and kept their diameters and path lengths (Grace and Llinás, 1985). In such cases, only the 3D spatial extent of the neuron would be affected but high spatial resolution sampling of the data would produce correct estimates of parameters such as path length along the neurites or neuron surface area.

When a large number of subtrees comprise numerous branches densely packed, there are alternative possibilities to connect neighbouring pairs of points. The cut ends of neuritic segments located at the tops and bottoms of adjacent sections to be merged do not coincide any more but are separated by gaps of various sizes (Figure 2.5).

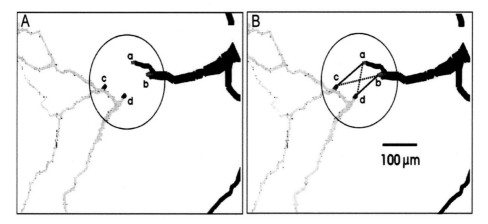

Figure 2.5 Gaps between adjacent serial sections. A: Zoom on pieces of neurites in two adjacent sections (dark and light grey) with cut ends a, b, c and d at the junction of two sections (circle) not coinciding due to instrumental and histological distortion. B: Possible connections between the cut ends are a–c, b–d, or a–d, b–c (circle). These connections are equally plausible and generate artificial links (worms). The larger the number of the worms, the larger the morphological noise. (From Kaspirzhny *et al.*, 2002.)

When connecting the pieces, several origin points can be considered as alternative merging partners. It may not be obvious to make a clear decision to choose one of the merging possibilities. Consequently, alternative topological variants may constitute equally plausible choices for the reconstructed neuron, creating the topological noise (Figure 2.6).

This topological noise linked to different possible choices is a component of our estimation of the morphological noise which evaluates all the 3D distortions included in the original data. However, the tools for evaluating the topological noise alone and for selecting the 'best' variant are difficult to design, since the original shape of the neuron in the brain remains unknown. These fluctuations in tree complexity reveal the existence of a topological noise which affects the topological description of the neuron: it is generated by the reconstruction process and combines with the metrical noise to produce the morphological noise.

2.5 Models of neurons

No-one has ever seen the original shape of a live neuron operating in a living brain and consequently there is no model a priori of the neuronal form. In physics, simplifying models have been useful in explaining large classes of phenomenon. If modelling is a strategy developed because complexities are an obstacle to understanding the principles governing the function, the neuron is a perfect example of

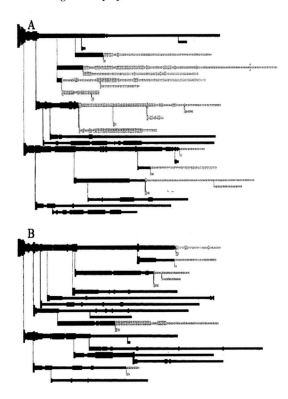

Figure 2.6 Topological errors introduced by metrical noise. Comparison of two dendrograms (A, B) obtained from the same dendrite of the same neuron digitized by the same operator but using two different acquisition systems. Topological differences between dendrites are grey in the dendograms.

extreme structural complexity to be tackled by modelling. The ideal and the reality seldom coincide and the resulting bias is usually unknown because the underlying assumptions go untested. The impact of bias on the accuracy of estimation and the validity of biological conclusions is also unknown. Keeping this warning in mind, modelling is the only available approach in the absence of experimental data allowing a detailed description of the neuronal system.

During the second part of the twentieth century, many books have discussed the advantages and the handicaps of the models. There is a wide variety of opinion over this issue leading to inappropriate attacks on, and defences of, neuronal modelling. Source books provide extensive bibliographies on the matter. An extensive bibliography together with original articles has been collected in the two volumes of *Neurocomputing* (Anderson and Rosenfeld, 1988). In 1855, Thomson (later to become Lord Kelvin) published his exposition of cable theory wherein longitudinal conduction in thin cylindrical elements was described in terms of one spatial dimension and time. Around 1900, several investigators admitted the applicability of Thomson's theory to core conduction in neurons. All important contributions to the understanding of electrical signal processing in dendrites have been based on this approach. Seminal books and reviews on these contributions are provided by outstanding contributors (Davis and Lorente de Nó, 1947; Rall, 1960, 1962a, b; Taylor, 1963; Harmon and Lewis, 1966; Rall, 1967; Rall and Shepherd, 1968; Rall, 1970; Jack *et al.*, 1975; Rall, 1977; Tuckwell, 1985; Macgregor, 1987; Durbin *et al.*, 1989; Rall, 1989; Holmes and Rall, 1992; McKenna *et al.*, 1992; Koch and Segev, 1999).

In the late 1950s, Wilfrid Rall, a physicist educated at Yale, proposed the application of the cable theory to dendritic arborizations (Rall, 1957). It was Rall who demonstrated that the time constant estimates found by Frank and Fuortes (1956) and by Eccles and collaborators (Coombs *et al.*, 1956) had resulted from misinterpretation of the voltage transient treated as a simple exponential. This assumption would have been valid only if the motoneurons were a soma without dendrites. Rall published a note in 1957 to establish this point and a detailed demonstration of his biophysical-mathematical theory in 1959 (Rall, 1959). The references to the introduction of Rall's theory in neuroscience are given in his autobiography (Rall, 2006). At that time, Rall played a crucial role in the understanding of the dendritic function by forcing researchers to re-examine their assumptions about the inexcitability of dendrites advocated by Eccles. In an interesting meeting of neurobiologists held in Amsterdam in 1959 (Eccles, 1960), Eccles presented his view on the properties of dendrites: 'The prolonged depolarizations that have been regarded as the characteristic dendritic response are merely the EPSPs that are produced just as well by the soma'. This conclusion deserved the attention of all neurophysiologists. Scientifically, it operated as a barrier to progress with few exceptions, particularly with regard to the opposing views of Chang expressed brilliantly in a Cold Harbor Symposium in 1952 (Chang, 1952, 2001) and some others (Bishop and Clare, 1952; Grundfest and Purpura, 1956; Bishop, 1958; Grundfest, 1958).

Ever since, all articles and contributions published by the numerous investigators studying neuronal dendrites contain a statement about the pivotal role of dendritic geometry for the transformation of spatiotemporal patterns of postsynaptic potentials into a time-structured series of action potentials. The amazing fact is that there is no comparison between the enormous amount of work dedicated to guessing electrical parameters by matching the theoretical predictions with the experimental data and the readiness to use simplified dendritic geometry (Redman, 1973; Fleshman *et al.*, 1988; Clements and Redman, 1989; Stratford *et al.*, 1989; Ascoli, 2002). Curiously, while stained neuronal structure can be directly measured in great detail with some confidence, the current choice of electrical parameters for constructing neuronal models is preferred, although they can only be inferred indirectly from measurements obtained by the microelectrode at a single site of the neuron. According to this approach, a plethora of unknown biophysical parameters offers a tremendous number of degrees of freedom available for constructing a model of the neuron. It seems that the emblematic tool of the electrophysiologists – the microelectrode and its recordings – cannot be dumped in favour of an approach consisting in direct precise measurements of the stained elements on histological serial sections.

There are studies using high spatial resolution reconstructions, however, that demonstrate the importance of local dendritic geometry. For example, they reveal that diameter changes and branch asymmetries displayed by the stochastic dendritic geometry determine the electrotonic structure of the arborization of single neurons (Bras *et al.*, 1993; Korogod *et al.*, 1994; Korogod, 1996; Carnevale *et al.*, 1997). Therefore, characterizing a neuron by its electrotonic structure depends strongly on the accuracy of morphometrical data obtained experimentally.

The qualitative or quantitative assessments provided by models rely on the type of approach chosen by the experimentalist. Currently, most modellers adopt a strategy of reducing the morphological complexity to 'equivalent cylinder' in order to generate 'canonical form', as described by Shepherd for constructing a computational neuronal model: *'A canonical model is the simplest type of a particular pattern of motif of neuronal structure and function that can represent a given neuron in computational form as a basis for simulating a functional operation or set of operation essential for that type'* (Shepherd, 1992; Shepherd *et al.*, 1998). The task is to identify the electrical properties that are critical for the particular input-output operations under study, in other words to be able to reproduce what is recorded by the microelectrode by a minimum number of compartments containing the minimum set of properties sufficient to capture the operations. Compartmental modelling is a similar method of coping with arbitrary geometries that is to divide the dendritic tree into a number of compartments, each of which is small enough to be considered as isopotential (Segev *et al.*, 1989). Most often, only two compartments are necessary to mimic microelectrode recording. So far, these strategies have provided most of the results obtained in modelling single neurons (see for references Durbin *et al.*, 1989; Stratford *et al.*, 1989; McKenna *et al.*, 1992; Stuart *et al.*, 2001).

In producing all kinds of output discharges resembling those well-known patterned discharges described by electrophysiologists, all the models elude a fundamental problem. They do not explain how the whole dendritic arborization contributes to the generation of the various adapted output discharges. Neither do they provide an understanding of the mechanisms that sustain the transfer function of all dendritic sites. For example, when Mainen and Sejnowski (Mainen and Sejnowski, 1996) show, using two compartmental models, that different dendritic geometry produce a variety of firing patterns in neurons that share a common distribution of ion channels, they stress the impact of dendritic structure on the pattern of output discharges. However, they do not provide an explanation for this difference.

This book proposes an alternative approach to the conventional models and introduces the notion of a functional dendritic space. We shall forget for a while the dogma of electrophysiology to concentrate on a detailed spatial description of the electrical states of all dendritic sites when the dendrites operate. By analyzing the electrical dendritic space in which all the signals are processed, we shall explore the spatial dimension of the transient events well known by electrophysiologists. We will demonstrate the mechanisms by which the operating dendrites decide, *in fine*, how the distributed synaptic inputs generate final various adapted output discharges. This original approach reveals the mechanisms by which individual dendritic geometry determines the sequence of action potential that is the neuronal code.

All neurobiologists know that a live neuron receives about 10 000 to 1 000 000 inputs which are distributed over its soma-dendritic membrane, which, in turn, contain dozens of different voltage- and time-dependent ionic conductances. These ionic channels interplay in the dendritic space leading to complex non-linearities in electrical behaviour. In principle, the electrical state of a neuron can be completely specified if its morphology and membrane properties are fully known. The only example described until now is the account of the electrical excitability of the squid giant axon by Hodgkin (1964). As for central mammalian neurons, unfortunately we must be content with very little, the vast unknown dendritic territory remaining a gamble on future research. Without this very minute knowledge, we are constrained to make assumptions and hypotheses. Conventional models have adopted a strategy that display single synaptic inputs in an arborization and simulate the recordings at single sites from the soma or some dendritic patches. In contrast, the approach implemented in this book considers that the whole dendritic arborization is homogeneously covered by defined synaptic inputs activated simultaneously with different intensities.

2.5.1 Uncertainties in the membrane properties of the dendrites

We acknowledge in several places of the book the fact that reconstructed geometries are known in fine detail unlike the electrical properties of dendritic arborizations that are known fragmentarily if at all. Neither composition of cocktails of membrane conductances nor their densities and dynamics are known for sure. However, we must specify these properties when performing any simulation. We are reduced to guessing them so they can be right or wrong. We adopt an experimental approach consisting of simulating the impact of a geometrical feature first

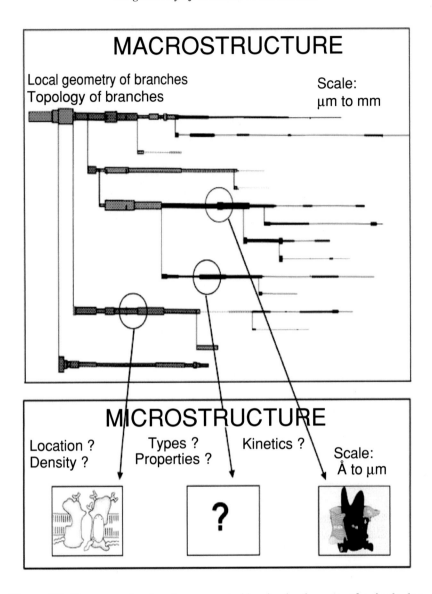

Figure 2.7 The macrostructure is represented by the dendrogram of a single dendrite extracted from a reconstructed motoneuron. Each branching point is shown as a thin vertical line. The macrostructure is a 3D object which is defined by geometrical parameters (length and diameters of branches) and its branching pattern (topology). The scale of observation is from mm to µm. Its inputs are distributed synaptic potentials along the branches. Its outputs are action potentials generated at the initial segment of the axon. The three circles indicate schematically dendritic sites from which a description of the types, location, density and properties of channels and receptors are, or should be, obtained to describe the microstructure represented below. They are toolkits of protein molecules. Their scale of observation is from µm to mm. The two scales of this functional unit explain why an immense territory of dendritic membrane remains unexplored.

on passive membrane properties. If the geometry-induced feature is observed in the simulation of the electrical structure of the dendritic arborization that receives single-site inputs, we conclude that this specific geometrical feature is responsible for the electrical effect. Then we test whether the geometry-induced feature is observed when the membrane is active with non-linear IV relation (Hodgkin-Huxley type or N-shaped) or when the true synaptic inputs are not single-site ones. For example, the simulations are performed with a membrane represented by spatial voltage profiles generated in response to tonic activation of distributed inputs. If the geometry-induced feature is again observed, we conclude that this specific feature is robust with regard to uncertainty of the membrane properties. A similar procedure is adopted to solve the problem of variability of the membrane parameters as we know that R_m changes as a result of ongoing activity. R_m decreases with increasing synaptic activation due to introduced synaptic conductances. The simulations are then performed at different values of R_m and we check whether the geometry-induced feature is observed whatever the values of R_m chosen in a given physiological range. Whatever the membrane properties, *the geometry determines the electrical states of the dendrites.*

In our simulations, we compute the electrical states of the arborization in different functional conditions and we observe the generation of unexpected patterned output discharges. Space and time of the phenomenon of the excited neuron are examined here for the first time.

We suggest considering the neuron as a macrostructure characterized by its 3D geometry made up of an organized microstructure specified by the macromolecules that populate its membrane (Figure 2.7). This functional unit is by now an immense unknown territory that plays the pivotal role in generating the neuronal code. Dendritic space is the focus of the following chapters of this book.

References

Anderson, J. A. and Rosenfeld, E. (eds.) (1988). *Neurocomputing: Foundations of Research*, Cambridge, Mass: MIT Press.

Ascoli, G. A. (ed.) (2002). *Computational Neuroanatomy. Principles and Methods*, Totowa, NJ: Humana Press.

Bishop, G. H. (1958). The dendrite: receptive pole of the neurone. *Electroencephalogr. Clin. Neurophysiol.*, **35**(Suppl. 10):12–21.

Bishop, G. H. and Clare, M. H. (1952). Sites of origin of electric potentials in striate cortex. *J. Neurophysiol.*, **15**:201–220.

Bok, S. T. (1936a). The branching of dendrites in the cerebral cortex. *Proc. Acad. Sci. Amster.*, **39**:1209–1218.

Bok, S. T. (1936b). A quantitative analysis of the structure of the cerebral cortex. *Proc. Acad. Sci. Amster.*, **35**:1–55.

Bras, H., Gogan, P. and Tyč-Dumont, S. (1987). The dendrites of single brain-stem motoneurons intracellularly labelled with horseradish peroxidase in the cat. Morphological and electrical differences. *Neuroscience*, **22**:947–970.

Bras, H., Korogod, S. M., Driencourt, Y., Gogan, P. and Tyč-Dumont, S. (1993). Stochastic geometry and electrotonic architecture of dendritic arborization of a brain-stem motoneuron. *Eur. J. Neurosci.*, **5**:1485–1493.

Capowski, J. J. (1989). *Computer Techniques in Neuroanatomy*, New York: Plenum Press.

Carnevale, N. T., Tsai, K. Y., Claiborne, B. J. and Brown, T. H. (1997). Comparative electrotonic analysis of three classes of rat hippocampal neurons. *J. Neurophysiol.*, **78**:703–720.

Chang, H.-T. (1952). Cortical neurons with particular reference to the apical dendrites. *Cold Spring Harbor Symposia*, **27**:189–202.

Chang, H.-T. (2001). Hsiang-Tung Chang. In Squire, L. R. (ed.), *The History of Neuroscience in Autobiography*, Vol. 3, p. 189–202, London: Academic Press.

Clements, J. D. and Redman, S. J. (1989). Cable properties of cat spinal motoneurones measured by combining voltage clamp, current clamp and intracellular staining. *J. Physiol. (London)*, **409**:63–87.

Coombs, J. S., Curtis, D. R. and Ecdes, J. C. (1956). Time courses of motoneuronal responses. *Nature*, **178**:1049–1050.

Czarkowska, J., Jankowska, E. and Sibirska, E. (1976). Axonal projections of spinal interneurones excited by group I afferents in the cat, revealed by intracellular staining with horseradish peroxidase. *Brain Res.*, **105**:557–562.

Davis, L. and Lorente de Nó, R. (1947). Contribution to the mathematical theory of the electrotonus. *Stud. Rockfeller Inst. Med. Res.*, **131**:442–496.

Durbin, R., Miall, C. and Mitchison, G. (eds.) (1989). *The Computing Neuron*. Boston, Mass: Addison-Wesley.

Eccles, J. C. (1960). The properties of the dendrites. In Tower, D. B. and Schadé, J. P. (eds.), *Structure and Function of the Cerebral Cortex*, p. 192–203, Amsterdam: Elsevier.

Elias, H. and Hyde, D. M. (1983). *A Guide to Practical Stereology*, Basel: Karger.

Fleshman, J. W., Segev, I. and Burke, R. E. (1988). Electrotonic architecture of type identified alpha-motoneurons in the cat spinal cord. *J. Neurophysiol.*, **60**:60–85.

Frank, K. and Fuortes, M. G. (1956). Stimulation of spinal motoneurones with intracellular electrodes. *J. Physiol. (Lond.)*, **134**:451–470.

Glaser, E. M. and Van der Loos, H. (1965). A semi-automatic computer-microscope for the analysis of neuronal morphology. *IEEE Trans. Bio-Med. Eng.*, BME-**12**:22–31.

Grace, A. A. and Llinás, R. (1985). Morphological artefacts induced in intracellularly stained neurons: circumvention using rapid dimethyl sulfoxide clearing. *Neuroscience*, **16**:461–475.

Grundfest, H. (1958). Electrophysiology and pharmacology of dendrites. *Electroencephalogr. Clin. Neurophysiol.*, **35**(Supl. 10):22–41.

Grundfest, H. and Purpura, D. P. (1956). Nature of dendritic potentials and synaptic mechanisms in cerebral cortex of cat. *J. Neurophysiol.*, **19**:573–595.

Harmon, L. D. and Lewis, E. R. (1966). Neural modeling. *Physiol. Rev.*, **46**:513–591.

Hodgkin, A. L. (1964). *The Conduction of the Nervous Impulse*, Liverpool: Liverpool University Press.

Holmes, W. R. and Rall, W. (1992). Electrotonic models of neuronal dendrites and single neuron computation. In McKenna, T., Davis, J. and Zornetzer, S. F. (eds.), *Single Neuron Computation*, p. 7–25, London: Academic Press.

Horcholle-Bossavit, G., Gogan, P., Ivanov, Y., Korogod, S. and Tyč-Dumont, S. (2000). The problem of morphological noise in reconstructed dendritic arborizations. *J. Neurosci. Methods*, **95**:83–93.

Horcholle-Bossavit, G., Korogod, S. M., Gogan, P. and Tyč-Dumont, S. (1997). The dendritic architecture of motoneurons: a case study. *Neurophysiology*, **29**:112–124.

Jack, J. J. B., Noble, D. and Tsien, R. W. (1975). *Electric Current Flow in Excitable Cells*, Oxford: Oxford University Press.

Jankowska, E. and Lindström, S. (1970). Morphological identification of physiologically defined neurones in the cat spinal cord. *Brain Res.*, **20**:323–326.

Jankowska, E., Rastad, J. and Westman, J. (1976). Intracellular application of horseradish peroxidase and its light and electron microscopical appearance in spinocervical tract cells. *Brain Res.*, **105**:557–562.

Kaspirzhny, A. V., Gogan, P., Horcholle-Bossavit, G. and Tyč-Dumont, S. (2002). Neuronal morphology databases: morphological noise and assessment of data quality. *Network*, **13**:357–380.

Kater, S. B. and Nicholson, C. (eds.) (1973). *Intracellular Staining in Neurobiology*, Berlin: Springer-Verlag.

Koch, C. and Segev, I. (eds.) (1999). *Methods in Neuronal Modeling*, 2nd edn. Cambridge, Mass: MIT Press.

Korogod, S. M. (1996). Electro-geometrical coupling in non-uniform branching dendrites. Consequences for relative synaptic effectiveness. *Biol. Cybern.*, **74**:85–93.

Korogod, S. M., Bras, H., Sarana, V. N., Gogan, P. and Tyč-Dumont, S. (1994). Electrotonic clusters in the dendritic arborization of abducens motoneurons of the rat. *Eur. J. Neurosci.*, **6**:1517–1527.

Kötter, R. (2001). Neurosciences databases: tools for exploring brain structure-function relationships. *Philos. Trans. R. Soc. Lond. B*, **356**:1111–1120.

Kravitz, E. A., Stretton, A. O. W., Alvarez, J. and Furshpan, E. J. (1968). Determination of neuronal geometry using an intracellular dye injection technique. *Fedn. Proc. Fedn. Am. Socs. Exp. Biol.*, **27**:749.

Ling, G. and Gerard, R. W. (1949). The normal membrane potential of frog sartorious fibers. *J. Cell Comp. Physiol.*, **34**:383–396.

Lorente de Nó, R. (1922). La corteza cerebral del rató. *Trab. Lab. Invest. Biol. Univ. Madr.*, **20**:41–78.

Lorente de Nó, R. (1934). Studies on the structure of the cerebral cortex. *J. Psychol. Neurol. Leibzig*, **46**:113–177.

Lorente de Nó, R. and Condouris, G. A. (1959). Decremental conduction in peripheral nerve. integration of stimuli in the neuron. *Proc. Natl. Acad. Sci. USA*, **45**:592–617.

Macgregor, R. J. (1987). *Neural and Brain Modeling*, London: Academic Press.

Mainen, Z. F. and Sejnowski, T. J. (1996). Influence of dendritic structure on firing pattern in model neocortical neurons. *Nature*, **382**:363–366.

Mannen, H. (1966). Contribution to the morphological study of dendritic arborization in the brain stem. In Tokizane, T. and Shadé, J. P. (eds.), *Progress in Brain Research*, Vol. 21A, p. 131–162, Amsterdam: Elsevier.

McKenna, T., Davis, J. and Zornetzer, S. F. (eds.) (1992). *Single Neuron Computation*, London: Academic Press.

Rall, W. (1957). Membrane time constant of motoneurons. *Science*, **126**:454.

Rall, W. (1959). Branching dendritic trees and motoneurons membrane resistivity. *Exp. Neurol.*, **1**:491–527.

Rall, W. (1960). Membrane potential transients and membrane time constant of motoneurons. *Exp. Neurol.*, **2**:503–532.

Rall, W. (1962a). Electrophysiology of a dendritic neuron model. *Biophys. J.*, **2**:145–167.

Rall, W. (1962b). Theory of physiological properties of dendrites. *Ann. N.Y. Acad. Sci.*, **96**:1071–1092.

Rall, W. (1967). Distinguishing theoretical synaptic potentials computed for different soma-dendritic distribution of synaptic input. *J. Neurophysiol.*, **30**:1138–1168.

Rall, W. (1970). Cable properties of dendrites and effects of synaptic location. In Andersen, P. and Jansen, J. K. S. (eds.), *Excitatory Synaptic Mechanisms*, p. 175–187, Oslo: Universitetsforlaget.

Rall, W. (1977). Core conductor theory and cable properties of neurons. In Kandel, E. R., Brookhardt, J. M. and Mountcastle, V. B. (eds.), *The Handbook of Physiology. The Nervous System. Cellular Biology of Neurons*, Vol. 1, p. 39–97, Bethesda: American Physiological Society.

Rall, W. (1989). Cable theory for dendritic neurons. In Koch, C. and Segev, I. (eds.), *Methods in Neuronal Modeling*, p. 9–62, Cambridge, Mass: MIT Press.

Rall, W. (2006). In Squire, L. R. (ed.), *The History of Neuroscience in Autobiography*, Vol. 5, p. 552–611, San Diego: Academic Press.

Rall, W. and Shepherd, G. M. (1968). Theoretical reconstruction of field potentials and dendrodendritic synaptic interactions in olfactory bulb. *J. Neurophysiol.*, **31**:884–915.

Ramón y Cajal, S. (1911). *Histologie du Systéme Nerveux de l'Homme et des Vertébrés*, Paris: Maloine.

Redman, S. J. (1973). The attenuation of passively propagating dendritic potentials in a motoneurone cable model. *J. Physiol. (Lond.)*, **234**:637–664.

Sadler, M. and Berry, M. (1983). Morphometric study of the development of Purkinje cell dendritic trees in the mouse using vertex analysis. *J. Microsc.*, **131**:341–354.

Sadler, M. and Berry, M. (1988). Link-vertex analysis of Purkinje cell dendritic trees from the murine cerebellum. *Brain Res.*, **474**:130–146.

Schierwagen, A. and Grantyn, R. (1986). Quantitative morphological analysis of deep superior colliculus neurons stained intracellularly with HRP in the cat. *J. Hirnforsch.*, **27**:611–623.

Segev, I., Fleshman, J. W. and Burke, R. E. (1989). Compartmental models of complex neurons. In Koch, C. and Segev, I. (eds.), *Methods in Neuronal Modeling*, p. 63–96, Cambridge, Mass: MIT Press.

Shepherd, G. M. (1992). Canonical neurons and their computational organization. In McKenna, T., Davis, J. and Zornetzer, S. F. (eds.), *Single Neuron Computation*, 27–60, London: Academic Press.

Shepherd, G. M., Mirsky, J. S., Healy, M. D., Singer, M. S., Skoufos, E., Hines, M. S., Nadkarni, P. M. and Miller, P. L. (1998). The human brain project: neuroinformatics tools for integrating, searching and modeling multidisciplinary neuroscience data. *TINS*, **21**:460–468.

Sholl, D. A. (1953). Dendritic organization in the neurons of the visual and motor cortices of the cat. *J. Anat.*, **87**:387–406.

Sholl, D. A. (1956). *The Organization of the Cerebral Cortex*, London: Methuen and Co. Ltd.

Smit, G. J., Uylings, H. B. M. and Veldmaat-Wansink, L. (1972). The branching pattern in dendrites of cortical neurons. *Acta Morphol. Neerl. Scand.*, **9**:253–274.

Snow, P. J., Rose, P. K. and Brown, A. (1976). Tracing axons and axon collaterals of spinal neurones using intracellular injection of horseradish peroxidase. *Science*, **191**:312–313.

Stratford, K., Mason, A., Larkman, A., Major, G. and Jack, J. (1989). The modelling of pyramidal neurones in the visual cortex. In Durbin, R., Miall, C. and Mitchison, G., (eds.), *The Computing Neuron*, p. 296–321, Boston, Mass: Addison and Wesley.

Stuart, G., Spruston, N. and Häusser, M. (eds.) (2001). *Dendrites*, London: Oxford University Press.

Taylor, R. E. (1963). Cable theory. In Nastuk, W. L. (ed.), *Physical Technique in Biological Research*, Vol. 6, p. 219–262, New York: Academic Press.

Tuckwell, H. C. (1985). Some aspects of cable theory with synaptic reversal potentials. *J. Theoret. Neurobiol.*, **4**:113–127.

Uylings, H. B. M. and van Pelt, J. (2002). Measures for quantifying dendritic arborizations. *Network*, **13**:397–414.

Van Ooyen, A., Duijnhouwer, J., Remme, M. W. H. and van Pelt. J. (2002). The effect of dendritic topology on firing patterns in model neurons. *Network*, **13**:311–325.

Van Pelt, J. (2002). Quantitative neuroanatomy and neuroinformatics. Editorial special issue quantitative neuroanatomy tools. *Network*, **13**:243–245.

Van Pelt, J., Dityatev, A. E. and Uylings, H. B. M. (1997). Natural variability in the number of dendritic segments: model-based inferences about branching during neurite outgrowth. *J. Comp. Neurol.*, **387**:325–340.

Van Pelt, J. and Schierwagen, A. (1994). Electrotonic properties of passive dendritic trees – effect of dendritic topology. In Van Pelt, J., Corner, M. A., Uylings, H. B. M. and Lopez da Silva, F. H. (eds.), *Progress in Brain Research. The Self-Organizing Brain: From Growth Cones to Functional Networks*, Vol. 102, p. 127–149, Amsterdam: Elsevier.

Van Pelt, J. and Schierwagen, A. (2004). Morphological analysis and modeling of neuronal dendrites. *Math. Biosci.*, **188**:147–155.

Van Pelt, J., Uylings, H. B., Verwer, R. W., Pentney, R. J. and Woldenberg, M. J. (1992). Tree asymmetry: a sensitive and practical measure for binary topological trees. *Bull. Math. Biol.*, **54**:759–784.

Van Pelt, J. and Uylings, H. B. (1999). Modeling the natural variability in the shape of dendritic trees: application to basal dendrites of small rat cortical layer 5 pyramidal neurons. *Neurocomputing*, **26–27**:305–311.

Van Pelt, J. and Verwer, R. W. (1986). Topological properties of binary trees grown with order-dependent branching probabilities. *Bull. Math. Biol.*, **48**:197–211.

Verwer, R. W. H., van Pelt, J. and Uylings, H. B. M. (1992). An introduction to topological analysis of neurones. In Stewart, M. G. (ed.), *Quantitative Methods in Neuroanatomy*, p. 295–323, New York: John Wiley & Sons, Inc.

Wann, D. F., Woolsey, T. A., Dierker, M. L. and Cowan, W. M. (1973). An on-line digital-computer system for the semiautomatic analysis of Golgi-impregnated neurons. *IEEE Trans. Bio-Med. Eng.*, BME-**20**:233–247.

Zsuppán, F. (1984). A new approach to merging neuronal tree segments traced from serial sections. *J. Neurosci. Methods*, **10**:199–204.

3

Basics in bioelectricity

There is no bioelectricity without space. To produce an electric field, electrical charges must be separated in space. The distance separating the charge carriers – the ions – on the neuronal membrane ranges between 6 and 10 nanometres. The charges are separated by the action of non-electrical forces that must be organized in space. Pump molecules embedded in the membrane operate by chemical binding and unbinding of the ions on the opposite sites of the membrane. The shape of the cell membrane together with the membrane material determine the membrane capacitance.

3.1 Ions as carriers of current

In neurons the currents are carried by ions flowing in the conductive intra- and extracellular media, the cytoplasm and cerebro-spinal fluid. The intra- and extra-cellular media are conductors of the second class, the electrolytes. The ions are elementary species of both charge and substance. Therefore, two driving forces move them: electrical and non-electrical, diffusive or chemical. Both types of forces occur due to special properties of the neuronal membrane separating the intracellular solution from the extracellular one. Electrical forces originate from the voltage difference (gradient). Diffusive forces are due to gradient of ion concentration. Ions change their spatial location also as a result of chemical reactions, e.g. with intracellular or membrane molecules. Main ion species carrying currents are sodium (Na^+), potassium (K^+), calcium (Ca^{2+}) and chloride (Cl^-). Each species has different concentrations inside and outside the cell. Normally, for sodium and chloride, intracellular concentrations are lower than extracellular, for calcium much lower, whereas intracellular concentration is greater than extracellular for potassium:

$$[Na^+]_i < [Na^+]_o$$
$$[K^+]_i > [K^+]_o$$
$$[Ca^{2+}]_i \ll [Ca^{2+}]_o$$
$$[Cl^-]_i < [Cl^-]_o$$

In other words, there is a transmembrane gradient of ion concentration directed inward for Na^+, Ca^{2+} and Cl^- and outward for K^+.

3.2 Selective ion permeability of neuronal membrane

The three known conditions for a current to flow between two points require: (i) a difference of electric potentials between the points; (ii) carriers, charged particles and (iii) conductive pathway between points. The presence of ions by itself is necessary but not sufficient for the current to flow. For generating a voltage difference between inner and outer sides of the membrane the separation of positive and negative charges between these sides is required. The charge separation is provided by transferring ions across the membrane either along or counter to their concentration gradient. The physical nature of these opposite movements is different as they are provided by different molecular machines inserted in the membrane, the *ion channels* and *ion pumps*. The charge can be separated if the ion carriers cross the membrane dissimilarly, that is if the membrane has different permeabilities for different ion species in different directions. Indeed, if the membrane did not have such *selective permeabilities*, then each positive ion crossing the membrane would be accompanied by a negative ion of the same charge to keep the electrical neutrality of electrolytes on both sides of the membrane. In reality, due to selective permeability of the membrane, e.g. in relation to K^+, when a K^+ ion is moved by a diffusive force from the inner side with greater concentration to the outer side of the membrane, then an equal uncompensated negative charge (carried by large organic anions) remains on the inner side. Both charges are now separated by the membrane and create the voltage difference between the 'plates' of the tissue capacitor. This is the transmembrane voltage, which, by the sign convention, is counted as the difference of potentials (E) between inner and outer sides of the membrane:

$$E = E_i - E_o \tag{3.1}$$

The electric field, thus created, tends to bring back the positive K^+ ion. The transmembrane voltage increases while the number of K^+ ions crossing the membrane along the concentration gradient exceeds the number of those returning by the electric field. When the outward and inward fluxes of K^+ equilibrate then the net flux and, correspondingly, the net current are zero and the transmembrane voltage established in this situation is the *equilibrium potential* or *Nernst potential*. Quantitatively, it is defined by the *Nernst equation* that for an ion specie k has the form:

$$E_k = \frac{RT}{z_k F} \ln \frac{[C_k]_o}{[C_k]_i} \tag{3.2}$$

where R is gas constant, T is absolute temperature, F is Faraday constant, z_k is valence of ions of sort k and $[C_k]_i$ and $[C_k]_o$ are, respectively, intra- and extracellular concentrations of these ions. For $k = K^+$ and Na^+, the valence is $z_K = z_{Na} = +1$, for $k = Cl^-$ $z_{Cl} = -1$, and for $k = Ca^{2+}$ $z_{Ca} = +2$, and the corresponding Nernst equilibrium potentials are:

$$E_K = \frac{RT}{F} \ln \frac{[K^+]_o}{[K^+]_i}$$

$$E_{Na} = \frac{RT}{F} \ln \frac{[Na^+]_o}{[Na^+]_i}$$

$$E_{Cl} = -\frac{RT}{F} \ln \frac{[Cl^+]_o}{[Cl^+]_i}$$

$$E_{Ca} = \frac{RT}{2F} \ln \frac{[Ca^+]_o}{[Ca^+]_i}$$

Correspondingly, in the total ion current conducted across each unit area of the membrane (current density J), one can distinguish the channel and pump component currents:

$$J_{ion}(x, t) = J_{chan}(x, t) + J_{pump}(x, t) \tag{3.3}$$

3.3 Ion pumps

The function of ion pumps is to move ions against their concentration gradient. This is the main force maintaining unequal concentration of a given ion inside and outside a cell. Naturally, such translocation of charged particles of substance requires energy, and the translocation is called *active transport*. The energy is consumed from chemical bonds of adenosine triphosphate (ATP) in reaction with adenosine triphosphatase (ATPase). The pumps are different types of ATPase specialized for transportation of different ions, e.g. Na^+/K^+ ATPase, Ca^{2+} ATPase. The pump current is generated by the so-called *electrogenic pumps*, which translocate unequal charges in opposite directions. For instance, during each reaction cycle, the electrogenic Na^+/K^+ pump translocates three Na^+ ions from the inner to the outer side of the membrane and two K^+ ions in the opposite direction. So, the net Na^+/K^+ pump current is outward.

3.4 Ion channels

The function of ion channels is to conduct ions along their concentration gradient. Such movement of ions is called *passive*, because this is simply diffusion, which does not require energy from any source. The ion channels are protein molecules spanning the membrane and forming a pore in the bi-lipid layer. The passage through the pore is not always possible. This depends on a conformational state of the channel molecule in which the gate of the pore is open or closed. The conformational states change stochastically and so the channels are open or closed, permeable for ions or not. The probability of transition between the states and the life-time of the open and closed states are important determinants of the ion conductivity of the membrane. Different factors influence the transitions. The channels are classified following the leading factor. If the leading factor is the transmembrane voltage, the channels are classified as *voltage-gated* or *voltage-sensitive*. If the state of a channel is determined mainly by binding to some chemical substance, e.g. neurotransmitter or a current-carrying ion, the channel is classified as *ligand-gated* or *chemo-sensitive*, or more specifically *calcium-dependent*.

An important property of the channels is their *selective permeability* to certain ion types. According to this property the channels are classified as *sodium channels*, *potassium channels*, *calcium channels* or *chloride channels*. However, some ligand-gated channels are permeable for more than one ion species.

The ionic current through the membrane unit area J is determined by the membrane conductivity G_m and the *driving potential* $(E - E_q)$, that is the deviation of the transmembrane voltage E from its effective equilibrium level E_q. The membrane conductivity is the sum of single channel conductances of all open channels present in the membrane unit. In the case of voltage-gated channels $G_m(E)$ is voltage-dependent. The density of the total local current $J_{ion}(E)$ is hence a function of the voltage E:

$$J_{ion}(E) = G_m(E)(E - E_q) \tag{3.4}$$

being the product of two factors, the total membrane conductivity $G_m(E)$ and the driving potential.

The total membrane conductivity G_m is the sum of the partial conductivities:

$$G_m = \sum_k G_k \tag{3.5}$$

The effective equilibrium potential E_q is a dynamically varying value which changes if, at least, one partial conductivity changes with the voltage (see below). Voltage dependence of an ionic conductance is determined by two opposite processes, activation and inactivation, described by the kinetic variables.

3.5 Voltage dependence of membrane conductance

The first factor in Equation (3.4), the conductivity $G_m(E)$, is often voltage-dependent. This property is due to the voltage dependence of a channel transition from closed to open state (*activation*) and back from open to closed (*inactivation*). In fact, there could be many conformational states; usually one is open and the others are closed. The so-called *kinetic variables of activation m and inactivation h* describe this feature of the ion conductance mathematically. Typically, the relevant equation has the following form:

$$G_m(E) = \overline{G_m} \cdot m^p \cdot h^q \tag{3.6}$$

where $\overline{G_m}$ is the maximum value of the membrane conductance, p and q are integer powers. $\overline{G_m}$ is the sum of single-channel conductances of all channels in open state. The product of kinetic variables $(m^p \cdot h^q)$ determines which proportion of the whole population of ion channels are currently open and therefore contribute to the actual membrane conductivity $G_m(E)$.

The kinetic variables m and h obey the ordinary differential equation of the same form:

$$dm/dt = (1-m)\,\alpha_m(E) + m\beta_m(E) \tag{3.7}$$

in which the backward and forward rate constants $\alpha_m(E)$ and $\beta_m(E)$ are explicit functions of E. These functions usually are phenomenological, obtained by approximation of experimentally measured relations on a certain class of functions.

3.6 Effective equilibrium potential of multicomponent ion current

The second factor $(E - E_q)$ in Equation (3.4) includes the voltage explicitly. Equation (3.4) gives the local current-voltage relation (*I–V* relation) which is a key characteristic of the membrane unit properties for understanding the biophysical mechanisms of all current transfers in a complex electrical structure. A well-known example of equilibrium potential is the resting potential of the membrane E_r, which is often used as a reference level, from which the transmembrane voltage is counted.

The total transmembrane ion current obeys the superposition principle. It is represented by the sum of the component currents:

$$J_{ion}(E) = \sum_k J_k(E) = \sum_k G_k(E)(E - E_k) \tag{3.8}$$

where each k-th component is characterized by the corresponding partial conductivity G_k and equilibrium potential E_k.

For the multicomponent current with different E_k, the effective equilibrium potential of the total transmembrane current is defined as a weighted sum of E_k:

$$E_q = \sum_k (G_k/G_m)E_k \tag{3.9}$$

3.7 Membrane capacitance and capacitive current

A thin insulator (the membrane matrix made of lipids) with adjacent conductors (intra- and extracellular electrolytes) forms a tissue capacitor with an admitted specific capacitance C_m ranging from 0.7 to 1 $\mu F \, cm^{-2}$ (usually the latter value is used in theoretical studies). Like solid-body (hardware) capacitors, this structure allows condensing of the charges of opposite sign on the two sides of the insulator. The difference here is that charges are ions and the 'plates' are liquid layers of electrolytes. Otherwise, the nature of electrical processes remains common. The condensed charges create an electric field, the intensity of which (the voltage difference between intra- and extracellular layers of electrolyte) is proportional to the charge density per unit membrane area. The charges deposited on one side of the membrane attract the charges of the opposite sign and repulse those of the same sign on the other side. This is because the electric field of the charges spreads behind the membrane. Conversely, removing charges from one side reduces the attracting and repulsing forces on the other side so that corresponding ions freely distribute by thermal motion between the juxta-membrane layer and the bulk of the electrolyte. An important feature of such redistribution of charge is that the ions do not cross the membrane and their 'coordinated movement' (the current) is due to remote action spreading across the membrane. Such ion movement is known as the *capacitive current*, which is related to the voltage change per unit time by the equation:

$$J_c(x, t) = C_m \frac{\partial E(x, t)}{\partial t} \tag{3.10}$$

This is the time derivative of the equation relating the voltage difference between the plates and the charge density per unit area of the plate in any capacitor:

$$Q = C_m \cdot E$$

3.8 External sources

The source function Equation (4.18) also includes the contribution to the total membrane current from an external generator (stimulator) $J_{st}(x, t)$. The charges are delivered from an external generator to a given part of a cell via electrodes. Depending on the 'stimulation protocol', there are generators of voltage or current. Time-courses of the stimuli are diverse: single or multiple impulses of different amplitude and duration, steady levels, ramp with different starting and end levels and different rates of change, sinusoidal or special complex shapes.

3.9 Local current–voltage (*I–V*) relations

3.9.1 Steady-state I–V *relations*

A useful characteristics of the membrane generators is the relation between voltage and current measured in the steady state, the *steady-state local current–voltage* (I–V) *relation*. The term 'local' refers to a membrane unit with homogeneous electrical parameters and without any lateral current between this and other units. The command steady voltage is maintained from an external generator (operational amplifier). From the generator output, a corresponding stimulating current I_{st} is applied via the microelectrode. In steady-state, the sum of these currents is zero:

$$J_{ion} + J_{st} = 0 \quad \text{and} \quad J_{ion} = -J_{st} = -E_{st} \cdot G_{inp} \quad (3.11)$$

Hence, the local ion current in this case can be measured as the inverse of the stimulating current at the output of the external generator. The pump component J_{pump} of the total transmembrane ion current J_{ion} (3.3) is small. If it is negligibly small ($J_{pump} = 0$), the ion current is determined by the channel current $J_{ion} = J_{chan}$. Until indicated otherwise, we use the simplest, index-free notation J for the total channel current as all other components of the membrane current are effectively zero.

The ionic currents crossing the membrane unit are fixed by the cocktails of membrane conductivities. The number of possible combinations of different conductivity types is huge and thus, the possible *I–V* relations are also enormous. However, it can be demonstrated that there are three major types of *I–V* relation, whatever the cocktails of the conductivities are: linear, non-linear with positive slope and non-linear with positive-negative slopes (Figure 3.1).

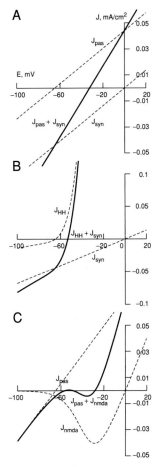

Figure 3.1 Three main types of the local current–voltage (*I–V*) relation in the membranes. A and B: Respectively, type 1, linear and type 2, non-linear *I–V*s both having positive slope in the whole range of the transmembrane voltages (abscissas, *E*, mV). C: Type 3, non-linear N-shaped with alternating positive and negative slopes in different voltage ranges. Exemplified are the membrane properties used in further simulations. Ordinates: *J*, mA cm^{-2} is the density of the total membrane current (solid line) and its synaptic and extra-synaptic components (dashed lines): (A) both components J_{syn} and J_{pas} are linear; (B) the synaptic component J_{syn} is linear and the extra-synaptic one J_{HH} is Hodgkin–Huxley type non-linear; (C) synaptic component through NMDA-type glutamatergic channels J_{nmda} is non-linear with the limb of negative slope and extra-synaptic J_{pas} is linear.

Linear I–V

Analysis of expression (3.4) shows that the local transmembrane current is a linear function of the transmembrane voltage when conductivity *G* is voltage independent. The plot of this *I–V* relation produces a straight line with a constant positive slope *G* which crosses the voltage axis at a point corresponding to the reversal potential $E = E_r$ where the current is zero (Figure 3.1, A).

Non-linear I–V with positive slope

When the conductivity depends on the voltage, $G = G(E)$, the I–V relation is non-linear and the slope varies according to the voltages. One example of this I–V relation is the non-linear steady relation between total current and voltage in the membrane of the giant axon of the squid. This relation includes sodium, potassium and leak currents and is described by the conventional Hodgkin–Huxley equation of excitable membrane:

$$J(E) = \overline{G}_{Na}m^3h(E - E_{Na}) + \overline{G}_K n^4(E - E_K) + G_L(E - E_L) \qquad (3.12)$$

The plot of this function has a positive slope in the whole range of physiologically reasonable voltages (Figure 3.1, B). It crosses the voltage axis at a single point which corresponds to the resting potential of the axonal membrane.

Non-linear I–V with negative-positive slope

One example of this type of relation is provided by a membrane containing synaptic conductance of inward non-inactivating current through voltage-sensitive glutamate-gated channels which are also sensitive to N-*methyl-D-aspartate* (NMDA). The cocktail of this conductance with the voltage-independent synaptic (AMPA type) and extra-synaptic conductances producing inward and outward currents respectively gives a non-linear I–V relation with a negative part of the slope (Figure 3.1, C). This N-shaped curve can cross the voltage axis in one or three points depending on the values of the conductivities.

3.9.2 Instantaneous local I–V relations

The steady-state I–V is informative but is an incomplete description of the electrical properties of the membrane. Additional important information is conveyed by the so-called *instantaneous* current–voltage relation. Considering the difference between the steady-state and the instantaneous I–Vs gives a more profound insight into the nature of electrical processes generated by the neuronal membrane (Khodorov, 1975).

The time-course of instantaneous I–Vs, e.g. during relaxation to a steady-state relation, is informative with regard to membrane properties dominating in the steady state (rest) and during generation of transients. A demonstrative example is the evolution of the I–V relation of the Hodgkin–Huxley membrane. The instantaneous I–V relation has a limb of negative slope and thus exemplifies the N-shaped relation.

This type of I–V is associated with the ability of the membrane to produce an auto-regenerative response, the action potential in this case. With relaxation to the steady state this limb gradually disappears and the ultimate I–V relation is non-linear with a positive slope. Such a relation indicates that membrane has a unique resting state with the voltage corresponding to zero total membrane current. This state is stable in the sense that after small perturbations (deviations from the resting potential), the membrane tends to come back to the initial resting state. In response to a stronger stimulus, the membrane changes its I–V to an instantaneous one and becomes able to generate action potential.

Reference

Khodorov, B. I. (1975). *General Physiology of Excitable Membranes [in Russian]*, Moscow: Nauka.

4

Cable theory and dendrites

A relevant mathematical tool to describe the bioelectricity in the neuronal dendrites is *cable theory*, which is based on application of the so-called *cable equation* to the *core conductor* model (Kernleitermodel) of the dendritic structure conducting currents and voltages. Exhaustive description of the cable theory and its application to analysis of electrical phenomena in the dendrites is provided in several excellent works (Taylor, 1963; Jack *et al.*, 1975; Rall, 1977; Rall and Agmon-Snir, 1999; Koch, 1999). In this chapter, the basics of this theory are given with accentuation of the issues important for understanding the material in the following chapters.

Cable theory requires *space* in which electrical parameters are distributed. The *dendritic space* is shaped by the membrane into a tube-like branching structure. The tube diameter ranges from several micrometres (or even a fraction of a micrometre) to several tens of micrometers in diameter and the tube length can read hundreds or even thousands of micrometres. These dimensions of the *dendritic space* are much greater than the thickness of the membrane across which the charges are *spatially* separated to create the electric field. What happens in the *space* along and over the membrane tubes? This depends on *spatial* properties of the electrical field in this larger domain. If the charge separation and the electric field produced by molecular machines is different at different locations in the cable, then electrical voltage occurs and the corresponding current flows between these locations. The routes in the *space* along which the current flows are shaped by the dendritic structure. We focus on the electrical events in the dendritic cables. The *space* we deal with is reduced to one-dimensional routes or lines along the dendritic cable, the dendritic paths.

4.1 Dendrites as electrical cables

Cylinder-shaped neuronal dendrites resemble branching electrical coaxial cables. Both obey the same laws of electricity physics and are described by the same type of the so-called *cable equations* mathematically. Like hardware cables, the dendrites have a conductive core enveloped with coaxial insulator and conductor cylinders. The dendritic core and outer conductive cylinder consist of cytoplasm and extracellular liquid solutions of ions. The insulator cylinder separating them is a thin plasma membrane that is a lipid bi-layer. This insulator is leaky due to specialized insertions permeable for ions. The cable equation is a parabolic-type *partial differential equation* describing electrical resistive-capacitive systems (circuits) with *distributed parameters*. The parameters characterizing the neuronal cable structures are the specific membrane capacitance and conductance (or resistance) related to the unit area or unit length of the membrane cylinder and the cytoplasm specific resistance related to the unit volume or unit length of the axial cytoplasmic core. For a cable of diameter d, the membrane capacitance per unit length c_m and that per unit area C_m are related via perimeter (πd):

$$c_m = C_m(\pi d) \tag{4.1}$$

Similar is the relation between the membrane conductance per unit length g_m and per unit area G_m:

$$g_m = G_m(\pi d) \tag{4.2}$$

The inverse values $r_m = 1/g_m$ and $R_m = 1/G_m$, i.e. the membrane resistance per unit length and per unit area are related inversely:

$$r_m = R_m/(\pi d) \tag{4.3}$$

The cytoplasm resistance per unit length r_i and per unit volume R_i are related via the cross-sectional area of the core $(\pi d^2/4)$:

$$r_i = \frac{R_i}{\pi d^2/4} \tag{4.4}$$

The parameters in Equations (4.1–4.4) are spatially heterogeneous and variable in time. They are then functions of one-dimensional space coordinate x counted along dendritic path and time t. The electrical state of a cable at each site x and at time t is characterized by the transmembrane voltage $E(x, t)$, the membrane current per unit area $J(x, t)$ or per unit length $i(x, t)$ of the cable. One more physical value, especially important to characterize the electrical communication (coupling) between different sites, is the lateral (core or axial) current i_{core}. Noteworthy, there are *sign conventions* which determine how the voltage and current should enter the mathematical expressions in order to correctly reflect the physical picture of the events. The transmembrane voltage E is counted as the difference of electric potentials measured on the inner E_i and outer E_o sides of the membrane, 'inside minus outside' (the signconvention 1):

$$E = E_i - E_o \tag{4.5}$$

It is known that the electrical potential is a physical value determined with accuracy to an additive constant, i.e. counted from any constant level. In neuronal cables, the transmembrane voltage is counted from the so-called *resting potential* E_r (for details see below):

$$V(x, t) = E(x, t) - E_r \tag{4.6}$$

It is convenient because E_r is often constant in time and homogeneous in space, which means zero derivatives, $\partial E_r / \partial t = 0$ and $\partial E_r / \partial x = 0$. Therefore the corresponding derivatives of $V(x, t)$ and $E(x, t)$ are equal:

$$\frac{\partial V(x, t)}{\partial t} = \frac{\partial (E(x, t) - E_r)}{\partial t} = \frac{\partial E(x, t)}{\partial t} - 0 = \frac{\partial E(x, t)}{\partial t}$$

and

$$\frac{\partial V(x, t)}{\partial x} = \frac{\partial (E(x, t) - E_r)}{\partial x} = \frac{\partial E(x, t)}{\partial x} - 0 = \frac{\partial E(x, t)}{\partial t}$$

The membrane currents per unit length and membrane area are related, like membrane conductance or capacitance, via the cable perimeter:

$$i(x, t) = J(x, t) \cdot (\pi d) \tag{4.7}$$

These currents are positive if directed outward (the sign convention 2).

Ohm's law relates the core current and the lateral voltage gradient:

$$i_{\text{core}} = -\frac{1}{r_i} \frac{\partial E(x, t)}{\partial x} = -\frac{1}{r_i} \frac{\partial V(x, t)}{\partial x} \tag{4.8}$$

The 'minus' sign in the latter equation indicates that the positive current flows in the direction of voltage drop (the sign convention 3) provided that the spatial domain is chosen so that the increment of the path coordinate ∂x is positive, i.e. counted as 'greater coordinate minus smaller.'

4.2 The cable equation

4.2.1 Mathematical expression and physical meaning

For a cable of a given structure, which are the voltages and currents in all sites x and in every moment of time t depending on the parameters of the cable and of the external actions? This is provided by the so-called *cable equation* for which a set of corresponding values $\{x, t\}$ composes a *spatio-temporal definitional domain*. A well-known standard form of the cable equation written in terms of $V(x, t)$ and parameters per unit length of the cable (see Rall, 1977) is:

$$-\frac{\partial}{\partial x}\left(-\frac{1}{r_i}\frac{\partial V(x, t)}{\partial x}\right) = c_m\frac{\partial V(x, t)}{\partial t} + \frac{V(x, t)}{r_m} \tag{4.9}$$

In the case of homogeneous and constant parameters, this equation contains factors having dimensions of time when multiplied by r_m

$$\tau_m = r_m c_m = R_m C_m \tag{4.10}$$

and distance squared

$$\lambda^2 = r_m/r_i = R_m d/4R_i \tag{4.11}$$

Corresponding scaling by λ and τ_m gives the dimensionless path coordinate and time:

$$X = x/\lambda \qquad \text{and} \qquad T = t/\tau_m$$

The cable equation in the dimensionless coordinates (X, T) is another standard form:

$$\frac{\partial^2 V(X, T)}{\partial X^2} = \frac{\partial V(X, T)}{\partial T} + V(X, T) \tag{4.12}$$

In the steady state when the voltage does not depend on time $V(X, T) = V(X)$, Equation (4.12) is reduced to:

$$\frac{\partial^2 V(X, T)}{\partial X^2} = V(X) \tag{4.13}$$

Below we consider more general forms of the cable equation and the details that are important for the analysis of the transfer properties of the dendrites. In theoretical studies of dendrites, we deal with analytical and/or numerical solutions of the cable equations. The properties of these solutions are considered as a more or less correct reflection of the properties of the neuronal dendrites. Interpretation and explanation of the dendritic properties in terms of properties of solutions of the equations require a clear understanding of the physical meaning of all terms of the equation and their impact on the form and properties of the solutions. The standard forms of the cable equation (4.9, 4.12 and 4.13) are most often sufficient. However, we shall consider some other forms with an emphasis on the different terms of the equation, their physical meaning and on their relevance to different aspects of dendritic functioning. The aim is to understand better the impacts of the membrane properties and of the geometry on the electrical processes that occur in dendrites that receive various input actions.

As already mentioned, at each point (x, t) of the spatial-temporal definitional domain, the cable equation relates the membrane voltages and currents. The equation is based on two main laws of physics: Ohm's law and the current conservation law. In terms of parameters per unit length, the cable equation is:

$$i(x, t) = -\frac{\partial i_{core}}{\partial x} = -\frac{\partial}{\partial x}\left(-\frac{1}{r_i}\frac{\partial E(x, t)}{\partial x}\right) \tag{4.14}$$

In the case of a homogeneous segment in which diameter d and hence r_i do not depend on coordinate x, the cable equation takes the form:

$$-\frac{1}{r_i}\frac{\partial^2 E(x, t)}{\partial x^2} = i(x, t) \tag{4.15}$$

Using Equations (4.4) and (4.7), the cable equation can be written for a dendritic cylinder of unitary area:

$$-\frac{d}{4R_i}\frac{\partial^2 E(x, t)}{\partial x^2} = J(x, t) \tag{4.16}$$

The cable equation, in each form, equalizes two terms, the *cable term* and the *source function*. They are, respectively, the left-hand and right-hand sides of Equations (4.15) and (4.16).

4.2.2 The cable term

The cable term is the left-hand side of Equation (4.15)

$$-\frac{1}{r_i}\frac{\partial^2 E(x, t)}{\partial x^2} = -\partial i_{core}/\partial x$$

and Equation (4.16)

$$-\frac{\pi d^2}{4R_i}\frac{\partial^2 E(x, t)}{\partial x^2} = -(\pi d)\partial i_{core}/\partial x$$

It expresses the increment of the core current in an elementary cable segment ∂x located at site x that is the difference between the core currents flowing into and away from ∂x. The difference of the core currents at x (partial space derivative of the current) is positive if the out-flowing current is greater than the in-flowing current and vice versa. This term determines which current remains available for the exchange between intra- and extracellular space at a given site after exchanging with the neighbouring sites. So, it is 'responsible' for the description of the way in which any given site of the dendritic cable is electrically coupled with the neighbouring sites.

Lateral current

The core current, Equation (4.8), flows tangentially or laterally, i.e. along the dendritic membrane. It is pure Ohmic current due to voltage difference between the given element ∂x and the neighbouring elements of the cable. By 'the sign convention', a positive core current flows in the positive direction of the x coordinate. It depends on both electrical and geometrical parameters of the core: the cytoplasm resistivity R_i and diameter d. Indeed, any dendritic segment communicates electrically with all other segments (parts) of the cell by exchange of the current flowing through the core. The 'sending' and 'receiving' parts work as the *source* and *sink* of the core current respectively. The *current conservation law* means that equal lateral current flows between the same parts on the other side of the membrane, in the extracellular medium. The communicating parts of the cell play the opposite roles. The site of the source of intracellular, core current is simultaneously the sink of the extracellular current and vice versa. However, these equal lateral currents produce significantly different voltage drops. The voltage drop inside the cell is much greater than outside. The reason is the much smaller cross-sectional area $(\pi d^2/4)$ of the core conductor compared to that of the extracellular space, while the specific resistance of the cytoplasm R_i and of the extracellular liquid R_e are nearly equal. For that reason, the cable equation very often does not include R_e.

Local balance of transmembrane and lateral currents

The cable equation, according to the current conservation law, at each location x equalizes the membrane current and the increment of the core current:

$$i(x, t) = -\partial i_{\text{core}}/\partial x \qquad (4.17)$$

This local balance of currents means that, at x, the core current increases or decreases depending on positive or negative contributions from the membrane current. The *sign convention* requires 'minus' in Equation (4.17): to provide a positive difference between the in-flowing and out-flowing core currents (increment), the membrane current should make a positive contribution, that means inward and therefore negative.

4.2.3 The source function: electrical properties of a membrane unit

The source function is the right-hand side of the cable equation:

$$i(x, t)$$

or

$$J(x, t)$$

that is the membrane current generated by the element ∂x per unit length or area of the cable at location x. This function determines the type of sources of the electric field in the nerve cables. Like in any other physical system, the electric field in neurons has two types of sources, called sources and sinks. The current streamlets originate from sources and terminate at sinks. The sign of the source function determines the source type. The source function determines also the nature of electric field sources. Specifically, they are determined by the two major components of the function, i.e. of the membrane current. In terms of parameters per unit membrane area, these are represented by components of the membrane current density:

$$J(x, t) = J_c(x, t) + J_{ion}(x, t) + J_{st}(x, t) \tag{4.18}$$

where $J_c(x, t)$ is the capacitive current due to charge redistribution without crossing the membrane, $J_{ion}(x, t)$ is the ion current transferred across the membrane, i.e. the transmembrane current, and $J_{st}(x, t)$ is the current from external sources, that is the current of charges delivered via intracellular and extracellular electrodes from a generator of current or voltage (a stimulator).

4.3 Additional conditions required for solution

To get a unique solution to the cable equation with either linear or non-linear source functions, one needs to know additional conditions. The cable equation is the partial differential equation of the first order in time t and second order in spatial coordinate x. Correspondingly, the required additional conditions are the *initial condition* and *boundary conditions*.

4.3.1 Initial conditions

The initial conditions are put on the value of $E(x, t)$ function over the whole spatial definitional domain at an initial moment of time $t = t_0$:

$$E(x, t_0) = E_0(x) \tag{4.19}$$

4.3.2 Boundary conditions

The boundary conditions are put on the values of the function $E(x, t)$ and/or its first partial space-derivative $\partial E(x, t)/\partial x$ at each point of the boundary of the spatial definitional domain. In mathematical physics, three standard types of boundary problem are considered, depending on what is defined on the boundary. In the first type of boundary problem, the values of the function are defined. In the second type, the values of the first partial space-derivative of the function are defined. In the third type (called also the *mixed boundary problem*), the linear combination of the function and its first partial space-derivative is defined. For the dendritic cable equation, the standard boundary problems have their own specificity. The boundary conditions are applied at the root and terminal tips of a dendritic arborization. Consider a single dendrite of finite length l.

The first boundary problem implies that the membrane potential is fixed to its resting value E_r at $x = l$:

$$E(l, t) = E_r \tag{4.20}$$

That is equivalent to zero deviation of the membrane potential from the resting potential:

$$V(l, t) = E(l, t) - E_r = 0 \tag{4.21}$$

This condition is similar but not identical to the standard 'open-end' boundary condition used in electric circuit theory.

The second boundary problem implies that, at $x = l$, the lateral (axial) current is interrupted by the impermeable tip membrane, that is equivalent to zero voltage gradient. This is the so-called 'sealed-end' boundary condition:

$$-\frac{1}{r_i}\frac{\partial E(x, t)}{\partial x}\Big|_{x=l} = 0 \tag{4.22}$$

In terms of $V(x, t)$ it is written as

$$-\frac{1}{r_i}\frac{\partial E(x, t)}{\partial x}\Big|_{x=l} = 0 \tag{4.23}$$

The third (mixed) boundary problem applied to dendrites is known as the problem with 'leaky-end' boundary condition. Physically, this means that at the dendritic tip $x = l$ the core current flows out of the cell through the leak conductance G_L. This current is proportional to the transmembrane voltage counted from the resting level (by Ohm's law) and is equal to the core current approaching the tip (current conservation law):

$$-\frac{1}{r_i}\frac{\partial E(x, t)}{\partial x}\Big|_{x=l} = G_L \cdot [E(l, t) - E_r] \tag{4.24}$$

4.3.3 Coupling conditions

Real dendrites are structurally heterogeneous. The two major types of structural heterogeneity are the change in branch diameter and the occurrence of branching points (sometimes called a *node of branching*). A branch having an abrupt change in diameter can be considered as *piece-wise homogeneous*, i.e. composed of connected homogeneous segments. Usually, the branches connected to each other at the branching point have different diameters. Consider a homogeneous segment of diameter d_0, from which homogeneous segments of diameters d_1 and d_2 emerge. At the connection point, there is a step-wise change in diameter, i.e. structural heterogeneity. The connected segments are coupled electrically, i.e. the voltages and currents in the connected elements depend on each other in a certain manner. This coupling obeys two laws of electricity, the *current conservation* and the *voltage continuity* laws.

Conservation of current

The current conservation law means that the core currents flowing in and out of the connection site are equal in the coupled segments. In other words, at the site of heterogeneity, the algebraic sum of core currents equals zero. This law means that the charges do not appear from nowhere or disappear, they are just redistributed between different parts of space. A well-known version of this law is *Kirchgoff's rule* used in electrical circuit theory.

Continuity of voltage

Consider two regions with a common border. The *voltage continuity* means simply that the voltage remains the same when the border is crossed between adjacent points in the two regions. These relations are expressed mathematically.

Coupling of unequally thick homogeneous segments

For the two segments of diameters d_1 and d_2 and lengths l_1 and l_2 such that the end of the first segment $x_1 = l_1$ is the origin of the second segment $x_2 = 0$, it is assumed that the path coordinate x is directed from the origin of the first segment to the end of the second segment and is indexed as x_1 and x_2 along the corresponding segment. This is the simplest example of piece-wise homogeneous dendrite with a stepwise change in the diameter. Consider the adjacent pre-step and post-step points $x_1 = l_1$ and $x_2 = 0$. The core current flowing from pre-step to post-step segment (or in the reverse direction!) meets on the border with a corresponding geometry-induced stepwise change in the core resistance $r_i = R_i 4/(\pi d^2)$ even though the cytoplasm resistivity R_i is the same everywhere. The current conservation yields equality of pre-step and post-step core currents at the common point of the two adjacent segments:

$$-\frac{d_1^2}{4R_i}\frac{\partial E(x_1, t)}{\partial x_1}\Big|_{x_1=l_1} = -\frac{d_2^2}{4R_i}\frac{\partial E(x_2, t)}{\partial x_2}\Big|_{x_2=0} \qquad (4.25)$$

The voltage continuity yields:

$$E(x_1 = l_1, t) = E(x_2 = 0, t) \qquad (4.26)$$

Coupling segments at bifurcation

Now consider a bifurcation in which the parent branch of length l_0 and diameter d_0 gives rise to daughter branches of lengths l_1 and l_2 and diameters d_1 and d_2. The path coordinate x is directed from the origin of the parent branch to the ends of the daughter branches and correspondingly indexed within each branch as x_0, x_1 and x_2. At the common point of the three branches, i.e. at the bifurcation node, the coordinates are $x_0 = l_0$, $x_1 = 0$ and $x_2 = 0$, respectively. The current conservation at the bifurcation node yields:

$$-\frac{d_0^2}{4R_i}\frac{\partial E(x_0, t)}{\partial x_0}\Big|_{x_0=l_0} = -\frac{d_1^2}{4R_i}\frac{\partial E(x_1, t)}{\partial x_1}\Big|_{x_1=0} - \frac{d_2^2}{4R_i}\frac{\partial E(x_2, t)}{\partial x_2}\Big|_{x_2=0} \qquad (4.27)$$

The voltage continuity at the bifurcation yields:

$$E(x_0 = l_0, t) = E(x_1 = 0, t) = E(x_2 = 0, t) \qquad (4.28)$$

4.4 Input–output (point-to-point) relations in dendritic cables

4.4.1 Attenuation ratios and factors

Voltage attenuation

In the dendritic cable, the voltage transfer between sites x_i and x_j considered as input and output, respectively, is characterized by the *voltage attenuation ratio* that is the ratio of (greater) voltage at the input to voltage at the output:

$$A_{ij} = V_i / V_j \qquad (4.29)$$

It gives the number of times by which the input voltage should be reduced in order to get the output voltage. The inverse value is the *voltage attenuation factor*:

$$a_{ij} = V_j / V_i \qquad (4.30)$$

which gives the proportion of the input voltage to be taken for getting the output voltage.

Current attenuation

The current transfer between input x_i and output x_j is characterized by the *current attenuation ratio*, which is defined similarly to the voltage attenuation ratio as the ratio of (greater) current at the input to (smaller) current at the output:

$$K_{ij} = I_i / I_j \qquad (4.31)$$

Correspondingly, the current attenuation factor is:

$$k_{ij} = I_j/I_i \tag{4.32}$$

Directional reciprocity of voltage and current attenuations in passive cables

In passive (linear) cables there exists the *directional reciprocity* between the voltage and current attenuations. This means that for any two sites in the cable, e.g. x_i and x_j, the voltage is transferred from x_i to x_j with the same attenuation ratio as the current is transferred in the opposite direction from x_j to x_i:

$$A_{ij} = K_{ji} \tag{4.33}$$

4.4.2 Transfer conductance and impedance

The *transfer conductance* is one more value characterizing the transfer properties of a cable. It is the ratio of the current at the input site x_i to the voltage at the output site x_j:

$$G_{ij} = I_i/V_j \tag{4.34}$$

The inverse value is the transfer resistance:

$$R_{ij} = 1/G_{ij} = V_j/I_i \tag{4.35}$$

Similarly the transfer impedance is defined, but it deals with the transient signals.

References

Jack, J. J. B., Noble, D. and Tsien, R. W. (1975). *Electric Current Flow in Excitable Cells*, Oxford: Oxford University Press.

Koch, C. (1999). *Biophysics of Computation: Information Processing in Single Neurons*, New York, Oxford: Oxford University Press.

Rall, W. (1977). Core conductor theory and cable properties of neurons. In Kandel, E. R., Brookhardt, J. M. and Mountcastle, V. B. (eds.), *The Handbook of Physiology. The Nervous System. Cellular Biology of Neurons*, Vol. 1, p. 39–97, Bethesda: American Physiological Society.

Rall, W. and Agmon-Snir, H. (1999). Cable theory for dendritic neurons. In Koch, C. and Segev, I. (eds.), *Methods in Neuronal Modeling. From Ions to Networks*, 2nd edn., p. 27–92, Cambridge, London: MIT Press.

Taylor, R. E. (1963). Cable theory. In Nastuk, W. L. (ed.), *Physical Techniques in Biological Research*, Vol. 6, p. 219–262, New York: Academic Press.

5

Voltage transfer over dendrites

Dendrites as electrical systems with distributed parameters differ from electrical systems with lumped parameters in an important aspect: any dendritic site can be considered as either input or output or both. In that sense, we deal with an electrical system such that the inputs and outputs are distributed in space, over the whole *dendritic space*.

The voltage is a standard and direct indicator of electric states. Similarity or dissimilarity of voltages reflects similarity or dissimilarity of electric states at different locations in space. The sign and magnitude of the voltage, that is the difference in the transmembrane potential between the sites, determines what electrically communicates with what and the intensity of the sent/received signals. The sites communicate by sending/receiving charges, i.e. by currents. The current flows in the direction of the voltage drop. Hence, considering the path profiles of the transmembrane voltage, one can see from where and to where the current flows in the given domain. Given the core resistance of the dendritic cable, the current between neighbouring sites is proportional to the voltage difference. Since one cannot 'observe' the path map of resistances, the path map of the voltages is informative, however not exhaustively. For an exhaustive characterization of the electric states and of the electric communication between sites over the *dendritic space*, a complementary map of the membrane currents is required (see Chapter 6).

5.1 Dendritic cables in the steady state

In the steady state, there are no temporal changes in voltage, voltage-sensitive conductance and current. The time derivatives of all values are zero. Therefore the capacitive current is zero. The cable equation is simplified:

$$-\frac{d}{4R_i}\frac{\partial^2 E(x)}{\partial x^2} = G_m(E(x) - E_r) \qquad (5.1)$$

In terms of voltage counted from the spatially homogeneous resting potential $V = E - E_r$:

$$-\frac{d}{4R_i}\frac{\partial^2 V(x)}{\partial x^2} = G_m V(x) \tag{5.2}$$

The spatial distribution and the time evolution of voltage along the dendritic cables is described by the solution of the cable equation.

5.1.1 Characteristic solutions to the passive cable equations

Infinite homogeneous cable

The characteristic solution to the cable equation describes the voltage distribution along homogeneous cables of infinite and finite lengths with standard boundary conditions. In all cases, the boundary condition at the origin $x = 0$ is fixation of the membrane potential at a certain level V_0:

$$V(x) = V_0 \qquad \text{at } x = 0 \tag{5.3}$$

A special case is the semi-infinite cable extending from $x = 0$ to infinity, which means no boundary. In such a cable, the voltage remains bounded however far away from the origin (when $x \to \infty$). This requirement follows the physical law of energy conservation: to create a non-zero voltage at infinite distance, the source should have infinite energy, which is physically impossible. Mathematically this condition is written as

$$V(x) \to 0 \qquad \text{when } x \to \infty \tag{5.4}$$

The corresponding solution to the steady-state cable equation is:

$$V(x) = V_0 \cdot \exp(-x/\lambda) \tag{5.5}$$

Finite cable with clamped end

For a homogeneous cable of finite length l with the boundary condition of voltage clamped to the resting potential at $x = l$, the solution is:

$$V(x) = V_0 \frac{\sinh((l - x)/\lambda)}{\sinh(l/\lambda)} \tag{5.6}$$

Finite cable with sealed end

For the similar cable but with the 'sealed-end' boundary condition at $x = l$, the solution is:

$$V(x) = V_0 \frac{\cosh((l - x)/\lambda)}{\cosh(l/\lambda)} \tag{5.7}$$

Finite cable with leaky end

In the more general case of a 'leaky-end' boundary condition with leak conductance G_L the solution is:

$$V(x) = V_0 \frac{\cosh((l - x)/\lambda) + (G_L/G_\infty)\sinh((l - x)/\lambda)}{\cosh(l/\lambda) + (G_L/G_\infty)\sinh((l)/\lambda)} \tag{5.8}$$

where G_∞ is the characteristic conductance defined below by Equation (5.13).

5.1.2 Input conductance of dendritic cable

Input conductance is a useful characteristic of a dendritic cable in a steady state. It is defined from Ohm's law as the ratio of the core current to the transmembrane voltage at the input $x = 0$:

$$G_{inp} = i_{core}(0)/V(0) \tag{5.9}$$

In all examples below the input voltage is the same V_0 as defined by Equation (5.3).

Infinite cable

From Equation (4.8), written in terms of the cytoplasm resistivity R_i and the voltage V counted from the reference resting level, the steady-state value of the core current at the input $x = 0$ is:

$$i_{core}(0) = -\frac{\pi d^2}{4R_i} \frac{\partial V(x)}{\partial x}\bigg|_{x=0} \tag{5.10}$$

The voltage in this case is defined by Equation (5.5) and its partial derivative at $x = 0$ is:

$$\frac{\partial V(x)}{\partial x}\bigg|_{x=0} = -(1/\lambda)V_0 \exp(-x/\lambda)|_{x=0} = -(1/\lambda)V_0 \tag{5.11}$$

Taking the ratio of Equations (5.10) and (5.11), we obtain the input conductance of the semi-infinite cable:

$$G_{inp} = \left(-\frac{\pi d^2}{4R_i}\right)\left(-\frac{V_0}{\lambda V_0}\right) \tag{5.12}$$

Substitution of $\lambda = (R_m d/4R_i)^{1/2} = (d/4G_m R_i)^{1/2}$ into Equation (5.12) gives the following expression for the input conductance of the semi-infinite homogeneous cable, which is the characteristic value often used in many other expressions:

$$G_\infty = (\pi/2)d^{3/2}(G_m/R_i)^{1/2} \tag{5.13}$$

Finite cable with clamped resting potential at the end

Taking the corresponding partial derivative of the voltage (Equation 5.6) at $x = 0$ and putting this into Equation (5.9) and using Equation (5.13) gives the following expression for the input conductance:

$$G_{inp} = G_\infty \coth(l/\lambda) \tag{5.14}$$

Finite cable with sealed end

Using the same procedure, but taking the relevant expression for the steady-state voltage (Equation 5.7) gives the following expression:

$$G_{inp} = G_\infty \tanh(l/\lambda) \tag{5.15}$$

Finite cable with leaky end

Finally, using Equation (5.8) and the same procedure as above gives the following expression for the input conductance of a homogeneous finite cable with the leaky-end boundary condition:

$$G_{inp} = G_\infty \frac{\tanh(l/\lambda) + G_L/G_\infty}{1 + (G_L/G_\infty)\tanh(l/\lambda)} \tag{5.16}$$

5.2 Voltage transients in dendritic cables

Dendritic cables are usually not in a steady state. The voltages, currents and conductances at different sites change over time. Ultimately, the electrical transients are the most interesting phenomena from the point of view of the dendritic functioning. Generally, they are obtained as numerical solutions to the non-stationary cable equations. Getting such solutions, especially in the case of complex dendritic structures with non-linear properties, is a rather complicated procedure. Cable theory allows some informative solutions in simplified cases of passive dendrites receiving certain, 'standardized' input actions.

5.2.1 Green's function and transient solutions

For the non-stationary cable equation in dimensionless coordinates:

$$\frac{\partial^2 V(X, T)}{\partial X^2} = \frac{\partial V(X, T)}{\partial T} + V(X, T) - \frac{I_{st}(X, T)}{\lambda c_m}$$

where $I_{st}(X, T) = \lambda \tau_m I_{st}(x, t)$ is the stimulating current, the *Green's function* or *impulse response* is $V_\delta(X, T)$, the solution obtained in a particular case when the stimulating current is an infinitely brief pulse, which deposits the charge $Q_0 = I_0 \tau_m$

at the cable input, $X = x/\lambda = 0$. For instance, in the case of infinite homogeneous cable with a standard 'boundary condition':

$$V(X) \to 0 \qquad \text{as} \qquad |X| \to \infty$$

the solution is

$$V_\delta(X, T) = \frac{I_0 r_m}{2\lambda(\pi T)^{1/2}} e^{\frac{-X^2}{4T}} e^{-T} \tag{5.17}$$

For linear cables, the impulse response allows one to build-up the solution to the non-stationary cable equation, which describes the response to the input current of an arbitrary waveform $I_{st}(T)$. The arbitrary input current is represented as a sequence of δ-pulses appropriately 'weighted' according to the command waveform. The composite response of the cable to such input is the superposition of the impulse response function and the input current. The response voltage $V(X, T)$ is the sum (integral) of the impulse functions generated by each individual pulse and appropriately weighted by the pulse. Mathematically, this is the convolution integral:

$$V(X, T) = \frac{\tau_m}{Q_0} V_\delta(X, T) * I_{st}(T) = \frac{\tau_m}{Q_0} \int_0^T V_\delta(X, T') I_{st}(T - T') dT'$$

where the symbol $*$ denotes convolution and τ_m/Q_0 is the scaling factor converting the voltage V_δ into an impedance.

6

Current transfer over dendrites

Currents flowing between dendritic sites redistribute charges over the *dendritic space*. The *spatial* maps of the net current are complementary to the those of the membrane voltage. The current density maps show contributions, positive or negative, of different dendritic sites to the core current flowing in the dendrites. In neurons, the currents are transferred by ions, which are not only elementary charges but also elementary amounts of substance. The current flow into or out of a unitary volume of the *dendritic space* changes the amount of substance per unit volume, that is the concentration. Both electrical and chemical signalling in neurons is concentration dependent. The well-known examples include the Nernst equilibrium potentials for the transmembrane ion currents, the concentration-dependent currents such as calcium-dependent potassium current, concentration-dependent ion pumps in the plasma membrane and in the membrane of intracellular organelles, and finally ion concentration-dependent intracellular biochemical reactions of many vitally important substances. Hence, the current density maps are necessary for understanding the contribution of the current flow and substance fluxes across the membrane to the dynamics of ion concentration over the *dendritic space*.

6.1 Charge transfer ratio

The *charge transfer ratio* also called the relative effectiveness of the charge transfer, was first introduced by Barrett and Crill (1974) to characterize the contributions from different individual dendritic sites to the total somatopetal current transferred to the soma. By definition, the charge transfer ratio T_{kj} is the time integral of the voltage V'_j produced at the reference point, x_j, i.e. at the soma, by charge injected at the point under investigation, x_k, divided by the time integral of the voltage occurring at the reference point when the same amount of charge is injected directly at x_j:

$$T_{kj} = \frac{\int_0^\infty V_j'(t)dt}{\int_0^\infty V_j(t)dt} \tag{6.1}$$

Since in a linear (passive) cable, the time integrals are independent of the time course of the charge injection, T_{kj} is defined also by the ratio of corresponding steady voltages:

$$T_{kj} = V_j'/V_j \qquad \text{where} \qquad V_j' = V_k/A_{jk} \tag{6.2}$$

Hence the value calculated for the relatively simple case of steady charge injection is equal to that for transient injection, and Equation (6.2) is valid in the more general case.

6.2 Somatopetal current transfer and somatofugal voltage spread

6.2.1 Theorems

The lemmas and theorem given below are used for obtaining relationships between somatofugal voltage and somatopetal charge transfer in the same arbitrary complex dendritic path domains (Section 6.3). The derivations are based mostly on the known steady-state solution of the cable equation, e.g. Equation (2.25) in Rall (1989), describing the distribution of electrotonic voltage along a cable of finite length, $\Delta x = l$, with uniform diameter, d, and with the voltage clamped to V_0 at the origin and leak conductance G_L at the end:

$$V(x)/V_0 = \frac{\cosh((l-x)/\lambda) + (G_L/G_\infty)\sinh((l-x)/\lambda)}{\cosh(l/\lambda) + (G_L/G_\infty)\sinh(l/\lambda)} \tag{6.3}$$

The leaky boundary conditions are taken since they can represent an arbitrary continuation of the path and, when necessary, be easily transformed to either sealed or open ends by taking the corresponding limit. Uniform segments of passive cable $[x_j, x_k]$ (Figure 6.1) were used to compose arbitrary paths (Figure 6.2) with elementary piece-wise uniform and branching sections (Figure 6.3).

For current injections, the input conductances to the ground at the extremes of $[x_j, x_k]$ are

$$G_j = G_{j-} + G_{j+}, \qquad G_k = G_{k-} + G_{k+} \tag{6.4}$$

where G_{j-} and G_{k+} are the boundary leak conductances, and G_{j+} and G_{k-} are the input conductances as seen from the origin and the end of the segment, respectively.

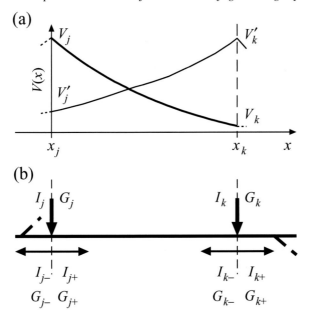

Figure 6.1 Electrotonic voltage as a function of x (a) for a uniform segment $[x_j, x_k]$ of passive cable, (b) when currents I_j and I_k are injected, respectively, at x_j and x_k, where input conductances to the ground are G_j and G_k, and input conductances met by the core currents, $I_{j\pm}$ and $I_{k\pm}$, are $G_{j\pm}$ and $G_{k\pm}$, respectively. (From Korogod, 1996.)

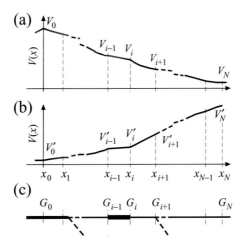

Figure 6.2 Steady voltage decay in the opposite directions (a, b) along an arbitrary piece-wise uniform route on a passive dendritic tree (c). G_i are input conductances to the ground at x_i ($i = 0, \ldots, N$). (From Korogod, 1996.)

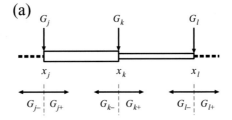

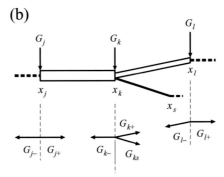

Figure 6.3 Elementary piece-wise uniform segments $[x_j, x_l]$ of the route shown in Figure 6.2 without (a) and with (b) side-branch offspring $[x_k, x_s]$ having input conductance G_{ks} for the core current at x_k. Other designations are the same as in Figure 6.1. (From Korogod, 1996.)

Lemma. *The ratio of the steady voltage attenuations, A_{jk} and A_{kj}, in the forward and reverse directions along a uniform passive segment $[x_j, x_k]$ is equal to the ratio of the input conductances to the ground at the end and the origin of the segment:*

$$A_{jk}/A_{kj} = G_k/G_j \tag{6.5}$$

Proof. Use Equation (6.3) for $[x_j, x_k]$ shown in Figure 6.1. The corresponding reciprocals of Equation (6.3) are the attenuation factors in the forward and reverse directions, respectively:

$$A_{jk} = V_j/V_k = \cosh(\Delta x/\lambda) + (G_{k+}/G_\infty)\sinh(\Delta x/\lambda) \tag{6.6}$$
$$A_{kj} = V_k'/V_j' = \cosh(\Delta x/\lambda) + (G_{j-}/G_\infty)\sinh(\Delta x/\lambda) \tag{6.7}$$

The ratio of Equations (6.6) and (6.7) reduced by $\cosh(\Delta x/\lambda)$ is

$$A_{jk}/A_{kj} = \frac{1 + (G_{k+}/G_\infty)\tanh(\Delta x/\lambda)}{1 + (G_{j-}/G_\infty)\tanh(\Delta x/\lambda)} \tag{6.8}$$

The ratio of the input conductances to the ground is

$$G_k/G_j = (G_{k-} + G_{k+})/(G_{j-} + G_{j+}) \tag{6.9}$$

Substitution of corresponding input conductances of the leaky segment written as Equation (2.37) of Rall (1989), namely

$$G_{j+} = \frac{\tanh(\Delta x/\lambda) + G_{k+}/G_\infty}{1 + (G_{k+}/G_\infty)\tanh(\Delta x/\lambda)} \qquad (6.10)$$

and

$$G_{k-} = \frac{\tanh(\Delta x/\lambda) + G_{j-}/G_\infty}{1 + (G_{j-}/G_\infty)\tanh(\Delta x/\lambda)} \qquad (6.11)$$

into Equation (6.9) gives Equation (6.8) and ultimately Equation (6.5).

Lemma. *The steady voltage attenuation along an arbitrary passive path, $[x_0, x_N]$ composed of N segments is equal to the product of the attenuations along all the segments $[x_{i-1}, x_i]$, $i = 1, \ldots, N$ composing this path:*

$$A_{0N} = \prod_{i=1}^{N} A_{i-1,i} \qquad (6.12)$$

Proof. Consider $[x_{i-1}, x_i]$ and $[x_i, x_{i+1}]$ in the path $[x_0, x_N]$ (Figure 6.2, c). The voltage attenuations along these segments in the forward direction (Figure 6.2, a) are

$$A_{i-1,i} = V_{i-1}/V(x)|_{x=x_i-} \qquad (6.13)$$

and

$$A_{i,i+1} = V(x)|_{x=x_i+}/V_{i+1} \qquad (6.14)$$

By virtue of continuity of the voltage, that is

$$V(x)|_{x=x_i-} = V(x)|_{x=x_i+} = V_i \qquad (6.15)$$

The product of Equations (6.13) and (6.14) is

$$A_{i-1,i} A_{i,i+1} = V_{i-1}/V_{i+1} = A_{i-1,i+1} \qquad (6.16)$$

Since the voltage is continuous in all x_i ($i = 1, \ldots, N-1$) including branching points, the same procedure being applied recurrently gives Equation (6.12).

Lemma. *The ratio of the steady voltage attenuations, A_{0N} and A_{N0}, in the forward and reverse directions along an arbitrary passive path is equal to the ratio of the input conductances to the ground at the end and the origin of the path:*

$$A_{0N}/A_{N0} = G_N/G_0 \qquad (6.17)$$

Proof. Consider two auxiliary cases. First, consider (Figure 6.3, a) the non-uniform non-branching path $[x_j, x_l]$ composed of $[x_j, x_k]$ and $[x_k, x_l]$ with G_j, G_k and G_l defined as in Equation (6.4).

By Lemma (6.12) the voltage attenuation along $[x_j, x_l]$ is the product of the attenuations along $[x_j, x_k]$ and $[x_k, x_l]$. Hence, the attenuations in the forward and reverse directions, respectively, are:

$$A_{j,l} = A_{j,k} A_{k,l} \quad \text{and} \quad A_{l,j} = A_{l,k} A_{k,j} \tag{6.18}$$

In Equation (6.18) factors $A_{j,k}$ and $A_{k,j}$, $A_{k,l}$ and $A_{l,k}$, respectively, are related to the same uniform segments. Hence by Lemma (6.5)

$$A_{j,k} = A_{k,j} G_k / G_j \quad \text{and} \quad A_{k,l} = A_{l,k} G_l / G_k \tag{6.19}$$

Substitution of Equation (6.19) into Equation (6.18) gives

$$A_{j,l} = A_{l,j} G_l / G_j \tag{6.20}$$

Since the above derivations do not depend on explicit expression of G_k, Equation (6.17) is also valid in the second auxiliary case (Figure 6.3, b), when the non-uniform branching path $[x_j, x_l]$ is composed of $[x_j, x_k]$ and $[x_k, x_l]$, with the side segment $[x_k, x_s]$ arising at x_k. The input conductances to the ground at x_j and x_l are G_j and G_l, defined as in Equation (6.4), whereas $G_k = G_{k-} + G_{k+} + G_{ks}$ additionally includes input conductance to the side segment as seen looking from x_k. Replacing G_{k+} by the sum $(G_{k+} + G_{k-})$ in Equations (6.9)–(6.11) results in the same Equation (6.20). Thus, this procedure being applied recurrently to all x_i from $[x_0, x_N]$ (whether they are branching or not) yields the proof.

Theorem. *The charge transfer function of an arbitrary point, x_k, of the passive cable in relation to any reference point, x_j, is equal to the reciprocal of the electrotonic steady voltage attenuation along the path leading from the reference point to the one under consideration*

$$T_{kj} = 1/A_{jk} \tag{6.21}$$

Proof. Use Equation (6.2) and Figure 6.1. For the voltages V_j' and V_j produced at x_j by the same currents $I_k = I_j = I$ injected at x_k and directly at x_j, Equation (6.21) holds. The voltage V_j' is related to V_k' by A_{kj} in the reverse direction:

$$V_j' = V_k' / A_{kj} \tag{6.22}$$

The voltages produced by the same current, I, at different injection sites are defined by the local input conductances to the ground:

$$V_j = I/G_j \quad \text{and} \quad V_k' = I/G_k \tag{6.23}$$

Substitution of Equations (6.22) and (6.23) into Equation (6.2), reduction of the equal currents and using Equation (6.5) completes the proof of Equation (6.21).

6.2.2 Path profile of the somatopetal current transfer

The soma is the natural common reference site, x_0 for all dendritic paths. When it is assumed to be isopotential with the whole cell input conductance G_0, then the injected current I produces the same voltage $V(x_0) = V_0$, at the root of every dendrite. Consider a dendritic site, x_d. According to Equations (4.29) and (6.17) the relative effectiveness of the charge transfer from x_d to x_0 is:

$$T_{d0} = 1/A_{0d} = V_d/V_0 \tag{6.24}$$

Provided that the voltages are produced by the same current, I, injected at different x, the relative charge transfer effectiveness of any dendritic site can be characterized in the same way and compared with those of other dendritic sites composing branches, paths and subtrees of the whole arborization. Since the somatofugal voltage, $V(x_d)$, is a continuous function of the path distance from the soma and the reference voltage $V_0 = $ constant, the relative effectiveness of the somatopetal charge transfer, $T_{d0} = T(x_d)$, defined by Equation (6.24), is also a continuous function on the same domain. The profile of $T(x_d)$ is completely defined by the corresponding profile of the normalized somatofugal voltage, $V(x_d)/V_0$, and the path behaviour of $V(x_d)$ induced by the dendritic geometry also represents that of $T(x_d)$. Correspondingly, the breaks in continuity of the voltage gradient induced at geometrical non-uniformities as a result of electro-geometrical coupling define the breaks in continuity of the path derivative, $\partial T(x_d)/\partial x_d$, that is, somatofugal decrease in somatopetal effectiveness.

6.3 Current transfer ratio for passive paths at different boundary conditions

The relationship between somatofugal voltage and somatopetal charge transfers (Equation 6.24) allows one to obtain current transfer ratios directly from the solutions to cable equations for different passive dendritic cables (Equations 5.5 and 5.8).

6.3.1 Uniform dendrite of infinite length

In the simplest case of an infinite length ($l \to \infty$), uniform (diameter D) passive (cytoplasm resistivity R_i, membrane resistivity R_m) dendrite, it follows from (5.5) that the transfer function is exponential:

$$T(x; R_m) = \exp(-x/\lambda) \tag{6.25}$$

6.3.2 Finite length dendrite with clamped end

Combining Equation (6.24) with Equation (5.6) gives the current transfer function for a finite length cable with the voltage clamped to the resting level at the distal end:

$$T(x; R_m) = \frac{\sinh((l-x)/\lambda)}{\sinh(l/\lambda)} = \frac{\sinh(L-X)}{\sinh L} \tag{6.26}$$

6.3.3 Finite length dendrite with sealed end

Combining Equation (6.24) with Equation (5.7) gives the current transfer function for the finite length dendritic cable with a sealed distal end:

$$T(x; R_m) = \frac{\cosh((l-x)/\lambda)}{\cosh(l/\lambda)} = \frac{\cosh(L-X)}{\cosh L} \tag{6.27}$$

6.3.4 Finite length dendrite with leaky end

Combining Equations (6.24) and (5.8) gives the following expression for the current transfer function for a finite length dendritic cable with a leaky distal end:

$$T(x; R_m) = \frac{\cosh((l-x)/\lambda) + (G_L/G_\infty)\sinh((l-x)/\lambda)}{\cosh(l/\lambda) + (G_L/G_\infty)\sinh(l/\lambda)} \tag{6.28}$$

Here R_m is included in λ and G_∞. Using notations $X = x/\lambda$, $L = l/\lambda$ and $B = G_L/G_\infty$, Equation (6.28) can be rewritten in a more compact form:

$$T(x; R_m) = \frac{\cosh(L-X) + B\sinh(L-X)}{\cosh L + B\sinh L} \tag{6.29}$$

6.4 Local electro-geometrical coupling in non-uniform paths

6.4.1 The sites of non-uniformity in diameter

Consider a segment $[x_0, x_2]$ of passive dendritic branch with a step change in the diameter at x_1 (Figure 6.4, b). The pre-step and post-step uniform sections, $[x_0, x_1]$ and $[x_1, x_2]$, have, respectively, diameters d_1 and d_2, and constant core conductances per unit length:

$$\sigma_1 = \pi d_1^2/4R_i, \qquad x \in [x_0, x_1] \tag{6.30}$$

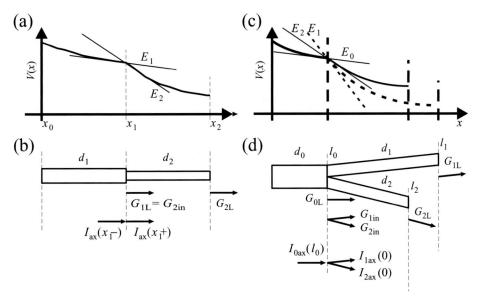

Figure 6.4 Voltage and gradient behaviour at the sites of step change in diameter (a) and bifurcation (c) shown in (b) and (d). Numbers 0, 1 and 2 added to subscripts mark the values corresponding to uniform segments. (From Korogod, 1996.)

and

$$\sigma_2 = \pi d_2^2/4R_i, \qquad x \in [x_1, x_2] \tag{6.31}$$

Assume that the voltage is clamped to V_0 at x_0 and decays towards the leaky boundary, x_2, with leak conductance, G_{2L}. At x_1 the voltage is continuous, $V(x_1-) = V(x_1+) = V_1$, the voltage gradient is discontinuous and the core current is conserved, which means:

$$\sigma_1 \mathcal{E}_1 = \sigma_2 \mathcal{E}_2 \tag{6.32}$$

where $\mathcal{E}_1 = \mathcal{E}(x_1-)$ and $\mathcal{E}_2 = \mathcal{E}(x_1+)$. As follows from Equations (6.30–6.32), the ratio of post-step to pre-step gradient at this site is determined by the purely geometrical ratio of the inverse square diameters:

$$\Psi_{21} = \mathcal{E}_2/\mathcal{E}_1 = (d_1/d_2)^2 \tag{6.33}$$

although the gradients themselves do depend on electrical parameters of the cable, boundary conditions and voltage.

6.4.2 The branching point

Consider a bifurcation node (Figure 6.4, c). Let the parent and the two daughter segments have the lengths l_0, l_1 and l_2 and the uniform diameters d_0, d_1 and

d_2, respectively. The corresponding constant values of $\sigma_i(x)$ are σ_0, σ_1 and σ_2. The voltage at the origin of the structure is V_0. The daughter segments have 'leaky' ends with the leakage conductances G_{1L} and G_{2L}. The steady-state voltage distributed along the parent segment is described similarly to Equation (6.3) with $G_L = G_{0L} = G_{1in} + G_{2in}$ now determined by leakages into the two daughter branches. At the node, the voltage is continuous, yielding equality of the pre- and post-node values:

$$V_0(l_0) = V_1(0) = V_2(0) \tag{6.34}$$

The condition of conservation of the core current written in a form similar to Equation (6.32) here involves three terms, $\sigma_0 \mathcal{E}_0 = \sigma_1 \mathcal{E}_1 + \sigma_2 \mathcal{E}_2$, from which it follows that:

$$d_0^2 \mathcal{E}_0 = d_1^2 \mathcal{E}_1 + d_2^2 \mathcal{E}_2 \tag{6.35}$$

It is noteworthy that the axial current and the voltage produced at the origin of each daughter branch are linked with the factor of input conductance:

$$I_{ax1} = \sigma_1 \mathcal{E}_1 = G_{1in} V_1(0) \tag{6.36}$$

and

$$I_{ax2} = \sigma_2 \mathcal{E}_2 = G_{2in} V_2(0) \tag{6.37}$$

The post-node gradient at the origin of a certain daughter branch may be related either to that at the origin of the sister branch, or to the pre-node gradient at the end of the parent branch. Consider the gradient $\mathcal{E}_1$. The ratio of the post-node gradients can be obtained by dividing I_{ax1} by I_{ax2} from Equations (6.36–6.37) and taking account of Equation (6.34):

$$\Psi_{12} = \mathcal{E}_1/\mathcal{E}_2 = (d_2/d_1)^2 (G_{1in}/G_{2in}) \tag{6.38}$$

Dividing Equation (6.35) by $d_1^2 \mathcal{E}_1$ with regard to Equation (6.38), one obtains the ratio of post-node and pre-node gradients:

$$\Psi_{10} = \mathcal{E}_1/\mathcal{E}_0 = (d_0/d_1)^2 G_{1in}/(G_{1in} + G_{2in}) \tag{6.39}$$

Reciprocally, $\Psi_{21} = \mathcal{E}_2/\mathcal{E}_1 = 1/\Psi_{12}$ and $\Psi_{01} = \mathcal{E}_0/\mathcal{E}_1 = 1/\Psi_{10}$. As follows from Equations (6.38) and (6.39), unlike at internal non-uniformity sites (Equation 6.33), the ratio of the gradients in different branches at the branching point is determined not only by the square inverse ratio of their diameters, but also depends on the input conductances to the daughter branches. This means that the electrical parameters of the membrane and the global geometry of the subtrees originating at the daughter branches may also influence the relative magnitude of disturbances of electrotonic gradients at the branching points.

6.5 Current transfer from distributed dendritic sources

According to cable theory (Jack *et al.*, 1975; Rall, 1989; Taylor, 1963), for any element x of uniform dendrite of diameter d the core current i_{core}, the gradient of the membrane potential $\partial E(x, t)/\partial x$ and the core resistance per unit length $r_i = R_i(4/\pi d^2)$ are related by Ohm's law (Equation 4.8). Consider Equation (4.14), defining the link between the core current and the total membrane current per unit path length $i(x, t)$, written in a slightly modified form:

$$\partial i_{core}/\partial x = -i(x, t) = -\pi d[C\partial E(x, t)/\partial t + J_{ion}(x, t)] \tag{6.40}$$

The increment (Equation 6.40) in the steady state ($\partial E(x, t)/\partial t = 0$) is defined only by:

$$J_{ion}(x) = G_m(x)[E(x) - E_q(x)] = G_m(x)E(x) - G_m(x)E_q(x) \tag{6.41}$$

Once the path profiles of the steady voltage are computed, the corresponding path profiles of $G_m(x)$, $E_q(x)$ and $J_{ion}(x)$ can be defined by Equations (3.5), (3.9) and (6.41). As follows from Equations (3.4), (4.7) and (4.17) in the steady state, the elementary contribution to the core current can be obtained from the path profiles of the total membrane current per unit area or per unit path length:

$$\partial i_{core}(x) = -\pi d J_m(x)\partial x = -i(x)\partial x \tag{6.42}$$

Correspondingly, one can obtain the total core current collected from any dendritic path l by summation (integration) of elementary contributions along this path:

$$I_{core}(l) = \int_l \partial i_{core}(x) = -\int_l i(x)\partial x \tag{6.43}$$

Equations (6.42) and (6.43) give absolute estimates of the current transfer effectiveness of elementary segment ∂x and finite length path l, respectively, for the case of distributed sources. Dividing the core current from an elementary source (Equation 6.42) or that from any sub-path l' of the path l by the total path current (Equation 6.43) gives the relative contributions to the total core current $I_{core}(l)$, which are estimates of the relative current transfer effectiveness of the parts of the dendrite with distributed sources:

$$\partial T_l(x) = \partial i_{core}(x)/I_{core}(l) \tag{6.44}$$

$$T_l(l') = \int_{l'} \partial T_l(x) = I_{core}(l')/I_{core}(l) \tag{6.45}$$

For branching paths, the contributions are computed according to the rules of conservation of the core current at branching nodes.

References

Barrett, J. N. and Crill, W. E. (1974). Influence of dendritic location and membrane properties on the effectiveness of synapses on cat motoneurons. *J. Physiol.*, **239**:325–345.

Jack, J. J. B., Noble, D. and Tsien, R. W. (1975). *Electric Current Flow in Excitable Cells*, Oxford: Oxford University Press.

Korogod, S. M. (1996). Electro-geometrical coupling in non-uniform branching dendrites. Consequences for relative synaptic effectiveness. *Biol. Cybern.*, **74**:85–93.

Rall, W. (1989). Cable theory for dendritic neurons. In Koch, C. and Segev, I. (eds.), *Methods in Neuronal Modeling*, p. 9–62, Cambridge, Mass.: MIT Press.

Taylor, R. E. (1963). Cable theory. In Nastuk, W. L. (ed.), *Physical Techniques in Biological Research*, Vol. 6, p. 219–262, New York: Academic Press.

7

Electrical structure of an artificial dendritic path

The mathematical tools described in the preceding chapters can now be applied first to simple artificial structures for the sake of demonstration of the electrical relations between proximal and distal dendritic sites. Studying these relationships means analyzing the electrical states of the sites. In a dendritic cable, the *local* electrical state, that is the *state of a site*, is characterized by the transmembrane voltage, current and/or conductance. A set of values of voltage (current, conductance) defined at consecutive sites along a path forms the so-called *path profile* of the corresponding values. It is graphically represented by a plot of these values as a function of the path distance from the soma.

A single dendritic path has a unique dimension measured in units of distance *along* the dendrite. Electrical relationships between all the sites situated in this *continuous* one-dimension space at shorter or longer distances from the reference point, usually the soma, provide a one-dimension representation of *the electrical structure of a path*. The electrical relation between *proximal* and *distal* sites is the only type of spatial relationship that can be assessed by the electrical picture of a single path. As a single dendritic path (Figure 7.1) is the most simple building block of an arborization, its study provides basic insights into the complexity of the dendritic structure.

In this chapter, the impact of a variation in diameter on the electrical structure of a single dendritic path is analyzed in detail. The simulated neuron has an axon represented by a non-myelinated proximal segment 200 μm in length and 3 μm in diameter, a cylinder-shaped soma (length 20 μm, diameter 22.5 μm) and a single non-branched dendrite of the same length, 780 μm, either uniform (Figure 7.2, A) or with a step change in diameter in the middle.

The simulations are performed in two conditions illustrated in Figure 7.2, B and C. The first condition corresponds to the experiments performed in modelling studies (Stuart *et al.*, 2001), which mimic a single-site input applied by a synapse to the dendrite, the voltage from this external source being transferred to the soma

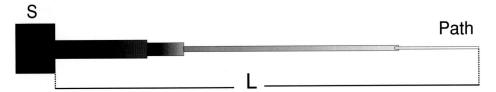

Figure 7.1 Schema of a single dendritic path which is a continuous structure from the soma (S) to the tip with two variables, length of the path and heterogeneous diameter.

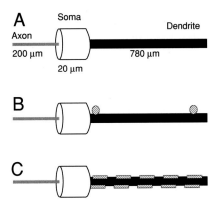

Figure 7.2 Schematic representation of the model neuron to study distal to proximal relations along a single path. A: Values of the geometrical parameters used in the model neuron. B: Single sites inputs (circles) at proximal and distal locations along the passive dendritic path. The specific membrane capacitance is $C_m = 1\,\mu F\,cm^{-2}$, the cytoplasm resistivity is $R_i = 100\,\Omega\cdot cm$ throughout the cell. The specific membrane resistivity R_m is variable. C: Multisynaptic inputs homogeneously distributed along the either passive or active dendrite. Specific electrical parameters are indicated for each case in the text.

and recorded there. This type of simulation experiment studies the relation between distal and proximal inputs. In general, the use of two compartments is sufficient although several compartments are also used.

The second condition (Figure 7.2, C) considers that a neuron never exists in isolation but is embedded in heavily interconnected neuronal networks that are active spontaneously. Therefore a spatially distributed, rather than single-site, activation of dendritic conductances is applied to the model. This condition is recognized as a more realistic input signal in many studies of input–output conversion in neurons, including simulations (Holmes and Woody, 1989; Abbot, 1991; Bernander *et al.*, 1994; Rospars *et al.*, 1996) and experimental research (Powers *et al.*, 1992; Powers and Binder, 1995). In some cases, activation of multiple discrete inputs can be a reasonable compromise (Rusakov *et al.*, 1996).

Based on laws of electricity physics, analysis of coupled electrical states of different dendritic sites and of changes in these states allows one to specify the relation between different sites and parts during spatial signal processing.

7.1 Electrical structure of passive paths with single-site inputs

Here we consider some simple examples of geometry-induced distal to proximal relations of electrical states along a simple path with passive membrane with type 1 *I–V* relation (Figure 7.2, B). Even though they are well-known, the smooth steady voltage distributions along uniform dendrites are computed as a reference for further consideration of electric disturbance at a local geometrical non-uniformity.

7.1.1 Path profiles of the membrane voltage

The case of different diameters and boundary conditions are shown in Figure 7.3, a and b. The smooth monotonic somatofugal decay of voltage has a greater rate along thinner dendrites. At a given distance from the soma, dendritic sites with different diameters display different voltages.

A step change in diameter, when large enough, causes an abrupt change in the voltage gradient (Figure 7.3, c, d). At the sites of diameter variation, the axial current meets a non-uniform conductance caused by an abrupt change in the cross-sectional area of the core conductor with uniform volume resistivity, R_i. Since the voltage is continuous and the axial current is conserved, the pre- and post-step voltage drops per unit length (the gradients) produced by the same current are inversely proportional to the core conductances of the unitary length sections of the adjacent pre- and post-step segments (Equation 6.32). Each of these conductances is proportional to the cross-sectional area of the corresponding uniform segment (Equations 6.30 and 6.31). Consequently, the gradients or the slopes of voltage decay are proportional to the corresponding cross-sectional areas, i.e. to the square diameters. Under both boundary conditions (Figure 7.3, c, d) when the pre-step diameter is greater than the post-step one, the somatofugal gradient increases (curve A) and vice versa (curves C and D). The greater the relative change in diameters (d_2/d_1), the greater the change in the slope of somatofugal voltage decay (curves C and D). In accordance with Equation (6.33), there is no dependence on boundary conditions, nor on R_m.

The information contained in the voltage path profiles provides the electrical picture of the dendrite, that is the electrical state of any site at any distance from the soma. Ohm's law says that the voltage drops in the direction of the current

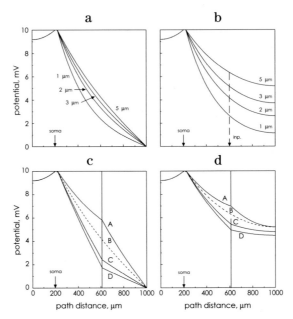

Figure 7.3 Somatofugal steady voltage distribution along uniform (a, b) and non-uniform (c, d) dendrites with open (a, c) and sealed ends (b, d). Location of the soma and the input of dendritic current are indicated by arrows. Diameters of uniform dendrites are indicated near the profiles in (a, b). Curves A to D in (c, d) correspond to different post-step diameters. Examples for the same pre-step diameter, $d_1 = 5\,\mu m$, and different post-step diameters, $d_2 = 3, 8$ and $10\,\mu m$ (curves A, C and D) in comparison to a uniform case (curve B $d_1 = d_2 = 5\,\mu m$). (From Korogod, 1996.)

flow. Hence, the plot of the voltage path profile indicates that the core current flows towards or away from the soma, depending on the direction of the voltage decay. The abrupt voltage drop observed when the current crosses the border between regions with different diameters, thus different resistances, is explained by the conservation law, which says that the core current is the same before and after such structural heterogeneities. According to Ohm's law in differential form, equality of the currents requires this abrupt change in the voltage gradient to keep the same core current. That the voltage gradient is a good sensor for revealing geometry-induced electrical heterogeneity of the dendritic core is thus demonstrated.

7.1.2 Somatopetal current transfer from single-site sources

According to the directional reciprocity of the somatofugal voltage profile and the somatopetal current transfer effectiveness (Korogod, 1996; Carnevale *et al.*, 1997; Koch, 1999 and see also Chapter 4), the pattern of the non-smooth somatofugal

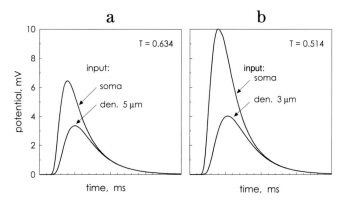

Figure 7.4 Excitatory postsynaptic potentials (EPSPs) at the soma in response to somatic and dendritic injections of transient synaptic current: plots (a) and (b) correspond to Figure 7.3, b. In the upper right-hand corners, values of relative effectiveness defined by the voltage-time integrals. (From Korogod, 1996.)

decay of voltage just described is identical to the path profile of the non-smooth decay of current transfer with increasing path distance from the soma.

In the same models, if we compare the transfers of steady currents to the transfers of transient currents, the values of T_{d0} can be computed for different sites on the dendrites and compared further. The calculations are performed in two ways. First, T_{d0} is calculated as defined by Equation (6.24) from the steady somatofugal voltage profiles e.g. those shown in Figure 7.3, b. Second, it is calculated from the original definition as the ratio of voltage-time integrals of the somatic excitatory postsynaptic potentials (EPSPs) produced by the same transient synaptic currents injected at the dendritic site under study and at the soma (see Figure 7.4). Figure 7.4, a and b shows the results obtained for the sites on single uniform dendrites of the same length but with different diameters. These plots correspond to Figure 7.3, b, in which the input site is indicated by an arrow. At sites equidistant from the soma, the relative effectiveness is greater for a thicker dendrite (diameter 5 μm) with sealed ends.

7.2 Electrical structure of paths with distributed tonic inputs

Distributed intrinsic current sources occur in passive linear or active non-linear dendrites when they receive tonic activation of multiple synaptic inputs over the whole membrane surface area (Figure 7.2, C). In active dendrites, such types of sources occur also when single-site inputs are activated. In these cases the charge/current transfer ratio (Barrett and Crill, 1974) is not an appropriate estimate of the transfer properties of different sites along the path under study. An adequate

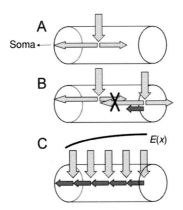

Figure 7.5 A: A single active input generates inward current which divides into the greater somatopetal and smaller somatofugal branches. B: Counter-directed branches of axial currents generated by two neighbouring synapses subtract and give an elementary net current directed to the soma. C: Repeating events shown in B give a chain of elementary somatopetal currents producing the membrane voltage $E(x)$ which drops in the direction of the current flow.

alternative is the universal estimate proposed by Korogod and Kulagina (1998b) (see also Chapter 4).

7.2.1 Voltage transfer from distributed sources

The universal estimate (Equation 6.42) calculates the contributions of each element ∂x of the dendritic path to the total current collected over the path receiving distributed excitatory inputs (sources), and transferred to the region of distributed sinks of the core current, usually the soma and the initial segment of the axon (Korogod and Kulagina, 1998b).

What is the physical picture of these events? It is illustrated by the explanatory Figure 7.5. Consider a dendrite with the membrane homogeneously covered by excitatory synapses receiving tonic activation of equal intensity (pre-synaptic firing rate). At each synaptic site, equal synaptic conductances are then introduced (Abbot, 1991). An input inward current of a certain intensity is generated at each site as this conductance is associated with depolarizing reversal potential (Figure 7.5, A). When this transmembrane current enters the core, it meets unequal input conductances in the somatopetal and somatofugal directions. The input conductance in the somatopetal direction is greater than in the somatofugal direction because the soma, having a relatively big volume and an attached axon, provides a much better leak at the proximal end than the thin distal terminals that have big resistances. Thus, the input current at these sites partitions into unequal lateral branches, the greater branch directed to the greater conductance, i.e. somatopetally.

Now consider two neighbouring synapses doing the same (Figure 7.5, B). At both sites, we have two branches of the core current, a greater somatopetal and smaller somatofugal. The unequal counter-directed branches of the core currents generated by these synapses subtract so that the resulting net current is directed somatopetally. Finally, consider a chain of neighbouring synapses again doing the same. The events near each pair are the same so that we have a chain of elements of the core current directed towards the soma (Figure 7.5, C). The superposition or the algebraic sum of the core currents at each site provides the net core current increment, positive or negative (decrement in the latter case). By the current conservation law, this equals the net local transmembrane current.

Hence, the principal structural asymmetry of the proximal and distal parts of a dendrite causes asymmetry of the lateral input conductances and inequality of the somatopetal and somatofugal portions of the core current, which is equal to the inward current at each synaptic location. This inequality leads to the occurrence of the somatopetal core current which receives contributions of inward currents from the distributed sources of tonically activated excitatory synapses. Here again, remember that the voltage drops along the dendrite in the direction of the core current flow. It means the occurrence of a dendritic depolarization that decays from the distal towards the proximal end attached to the soma.

The purpose of such a schematic explanation is to facilitate the understanding of the complex events occurring in the following specific examples, when dendritic voltage, conductance and current are computed along the path. Consider a finite-length uniform dendrite receiving tonic activation of homogeneously distributed synaptic inputs. Its membrane properties are also uniform and are defined by the corresponding I–V relation. First, we consider the cases when the I–V relation has positive slope and is linear (type 1) or non-linear, the Hodgkin–Huxley membrane (type 2) (Figure 3.1, A or B).

7.2.2 Membrane I–V relation with positive slope

Compare two artificial neurons of the same morphology (see insert in Figure 7.6, b) like that described above (see Section 7.1). In both models, the soma and axon have identical passive membrane properties (conductivity $G_p = 0.677\,\mathrm{mS\,cm^{-2}}$ associated with the equilibrium resting potential $E_p = -65\,\mathrm{mV}$). However, the membrane properties of their dendrites differ. One is passive with $G_p = 0.0677\,\mathrm{mS\,cm^{-2}}$, and $E_p = -65\,\mathrm{mV}$ (Figure 7.6, a, c), and the other one is active with the same $\mathrm{Na^+, K^+}$ and leak conductances as the conventional Hodgkin–Huxley model (Figure 7.6, b, d) but with 10 times lower values to represent a lower channel density in the dendrites than in the soma (Katz and Miledi, 1963; Clements and Redman, 1989). The common feature of both dendrites is that their membrane I–V relations have

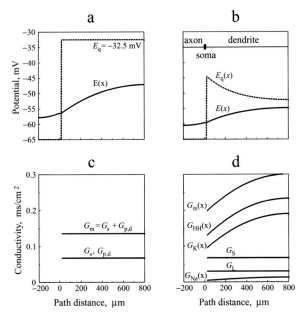

Figure 7.6 Path profiles of the membrane potentials and conductivities resulting from steady uniform activation of excitatory synaptic inputs distributed along a homogeneous dendrite with passive (a, c) or active (b, d) extra-synaptic membrane (simulated neuron shown in insert in b); a, b: transmembrane potential $E(x)$ (solid lines) and effective equilibrium potential of the total transmembrane current $E_q(x)$; c: homogeneous total membrane conductivity G_m and its equal partial conductivities of synaptic and passive extra-synaptic dendritic membrane G_s, $G_{p,d}$, d: non-homogeneous total membrane conductivity $G_m(x)$ and homogeneous voltage independent G_s, G_L components. $G_{HH}(x) = G_{Na}(x) + G_K(x) + G_L$ is non-homogeneous conductivity of the active extra-synaptic membrane of the dendrite. (From Korogod and Kulagina, 1998b.)

a positive slope over the whole range of voltages, but are linear in one case and non-linear in the other (Figure 3.1, A and B).

In the initial steady state, the path profile of the transmembrane potential and the equilibrium potential of the total transmembrane current are equal and uniform, $E = E_q = -65$ mV over the entire neuron. Introducing a steady uniform synaptic conductivity $G_s = 0.0677$ mS cm^{-2} (Figure 7.6, c, d) after relaxation of the transients leads ultimately to steady depolarization shifts of the transmembrane potential $E(x)$ and of the effective equilibrium potential of the total transmembrane current $E_q(x)$ (Figure 7.6, a, b, solid and dashed lines, respectively).

Consider the path distributions $E(x)$ and $E_q(x)$ produced by the same uniform activation of excitatory synaptic conductances along passive and active dendrites (Figure 7.6, a, b, solid lines). In both dendrites, the depolarization $E(x)$ is spatially inhomogeneous. It is highest at the distal end of the dendrite

($x = 800$ μm) and decays towards the soma ($x = 0$) and further to the distal end of the axon ($x = -200$ μm). The axo-somatic part of the path profile $E(x)$ is concave, and the dendritic part is convex. The path gradient (the slope of the path profile) of the transmembrane potential is positive along the dendrite and negative along the axon (note negative path coordinates of the axo-somatic part in Figure 7.6, a, b) and decreases with increasing path distance from the soma. The depolarization and its longitudinal gradient are greater when the dendritic membrane is passive (Figure 7.6, a, b, solid lines). The effective equilibrium potential $E_q(x)$ remains at the same uniform level -65 mV in the soma and axon, but changes in the dendrite depending on the properties of the extra-synaptic membrane. In the passive dendrite, it is shifted to uniform depolarization at $E_q = -32.5$ mV. In the active dendrite, $E_q(x)$ is also shifted to depolarization, but non-uniformly. The depolarization $E_q(x)$ is maximal at the proximal end of the dendrite and decays with increasing path distance from the soma.

The vertical deviation of the solid line from the dashed line in Figure 7.6, a and b defines the difference between the membrane potential $E(x)$ and the effective equilibrium potential $E_q(x)$, that is the driving potential $E(x) - E_q(x)$, of the total transmembrane current $J_m(x)$ (see below). With such path profiles of $E(x)$ and $E_q(x)$, the driving potential $E(x) - E_q(x)$ is negative in the dendrite and positive in the axo-somatic part. The absolute value of the driving potential decreases with increasing path distance from the soma. In the dendrite, the decrease is greater when its extra-synaptic membrane is active (Hodgkin–Huxley type).

Path profiles of total and partial membrane conductances

Path profiles of the total and partial membrane conductances are sensible descriptors of the electrical structure of the dendrites in two respects. First, they explain the shape of the path profiles of the effective equilibrium potential $E_q(x)$ (Figure 7.6, a, b, dashed lines). Second, they define the path profiles of the density of the total membrane current $J_m(x)$ and its components (see below, Figure 7.7, a, b). According to Equation (3.9), the effective equilibrium potential of the total transmembrane current is defined as the weighted sum of the partial equilibrium (reversal) potentials of the component currents. For each, the weighting factor is a proportion of a given partial conductivity in the total membrane conductivity.

In the passive dendrite, both synaptic G_s and extra-synaptic $G_{p,d}$ conductivities are voltage-independent equal and spatially homogeneous (overlapping horizontal lines in Figure 7.6, c) and so is their sum $G_m = G_s + G_{p,d}$ (in Figure 7.6, c, parallel horizontal line). Correspondingly, the weighting factors G_s/G_m and $G_{p,d}/G_m$ are spatially homogeneous and equal to 0.5, and so is the sum of the weighted equilibrium potentials of the passive membrane and synaptic currents

(Equation 3.9). This explains the spatially homogeneous path profile of E_q along the passive dendrite (Figure 7.6, a, dashed line).

In the active dendrite, the extra-synaptic dendritic conductances are voltage-dependent. They react to spatially inhomogeneous transmembrane voltage and, although their densities (maximum values) are homogeneous, the activation levels are not. Path distributions of the dendritic conductivities (Figure 7.6, d) show that although the synaptic conductivity G_s is uniform, the total membrane conductivity $G_m(x)$ and its main component, the conductivity of the active extra-synaptic membrane $G_{HH}(x)$, increases with path distance from the soma following the transmembrane depolarization $E(x)$ (Figure 7.6, b). The main contribution to this change in $G_{HH}(x)$ and thus $G_m(x)$ comes from an increase in non-inactivating potassium conductivity $G_K(x)$ associated with the hyperpolarization equilibrium potential E_K. The contribution from the inactivating sodium conductivity $G_{Na}(x)$ associated with the depolarization equilibrium potential E_{Na} is about one order of magnitude lower than that from $G_K(x)$. Increasing weight $G_K(x)/G_m(x)$ of the hyperpolarizing potassium potential E_K and decreasing weights of the depolarizing potentials make the effective equilibrium potential $E_q(x)$ of the total dendritic current less depolarized at greater path distances x from the soma.

This path profile of the transmembrane voltage defines the direction and the intensity of the core current. In the dendrite, the core current is somatopetal and its intensity increases towards the soma. In the axo-somatic part of the neuron, the core current is somatofugal and its intensity decreases with increasing path distance (Figure 7.7, c, d).

7.2.3 Current transfer from distributed sources

For electrophysiologists, the question of how to distinguish the contributions of the different dendritic elements to the net current delivered to the soma remains unsolved. This critical problem can now be considered by analyzing the path profiles of the total transmembrane current density per unit area in the passive and active dendrites shown in Figure 7.7, a, b. Our tools are Equations (6.40–6.42). Corresponding to the driving potentials, the current is negative (inward) in the dendritic part and positive (outward) in the axo-somatic part. The density of the dendritic current decreases with path distance from the soma. The current loss through the unit membrane area is the highest in the soma and decreases towards the distal end of the axon.

The plots of the increment of the core current as a function of the path distance from the soma are shown in Figure 7.7, c, d. The advantage of this presentation is that the area between the current plot and zero axis on any path segment defines directly the net core current collected from or consumed in this segment.

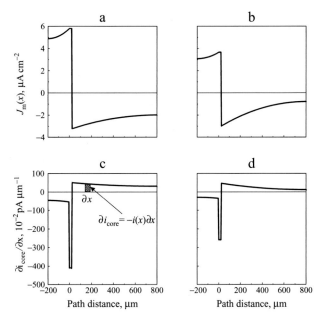

Figure 7.7 Total membrane current density per unit area (a, b) and increment of the core current per unit path length (c, d) as a function of path distance from the soma as a result of the steady uniform activation of excitatory synaptic conductances of the uniform dendrite with passive (a, c) and active (b, d) extra-synaptic membranes in the same neuron as in Figure 7.6. Shaded area in c shows the current collected from the path element ∂x. (From Korogod and Kulagina, 1998b.)

Figure 7.7, c, d, shows that the contribution to the core current is made only by the dendritic elements where the current production by the membrane generators $G_m(x) \cdot E_q(x)$ dominates over the current loss $G_m(x) \cdot E(x)$ through the load $G_m(x)$. The elementary contribution $\partial i_{core}(x) = -i(x)\partial x$ decreases with increasing path distance x from the soma in both passive and active dendrites. The passive soma and axon consume the core current delivered from the dendrite. The consumption has a prominent peak in the soma, is much lower in the axon and decays gradually along the homogeneous axon.

7.2.4 Membrane I–V relation with negative-positive slope

It is known that the N-shaped *I–V* relation (type 3, Figure 3.1) is provided by the contribution of a non-inactivating or slow inactivating depolarizing (inward) current, like the persistent sodium current or L-type calcium current through extra-synaptic voltage-gated channels, or the current through glutamatergic synaptic channels of a special type sensitive to *N*-methyl-D-aspartate (NMDA-type current). The latter is used here, as it is the minimum sufficient to provide the electrical bistability of the dendritic membrane (Korogod and Kulagina, 1998a). It illustrates the biophysical basis for the hypothesis that the persistent inward current can make distal dendrites more or less effective than proximal dendrites in the somatopetal current transfer from distributed excitatory inputs, due to voltage-dependent amplification of tonic synaptic currents (Schwindt and Crill, 1980; Bernander *et al.*, 1994). It shows that the distal dendritic 'dominance' or 'surrender' depends on the level and inhomogeneity of postsynaptic depolarization in an active dendrite. It is possible when the depolarization level is within the range of the negative slope of the membrane *I–V* relation.

The study of the electrical structure of a dendritic path which is electrically bistable provides a deeper insight into the mechanisms by which local membrane properties rule the comparative effectiveness of distal versus proximal sites (see Chapter 6).

To facilitate the comparison with the previously described models, the simulated neuron has the same morphology as in Figure 7.2, C. To highlight the intrinsic dendritic mechanisms, a constant leak conductance is kept at the proximal end of the dendrite with a sealed distal end. For that, the axo-somatic membrane is again assumed to be passive with specific conductivity $G_{p,s} = 0.677 \, \text{mS cm}^{-2}$ and reversal potential $E_p = -65 \, \text{mV}$. Numerically, this conductivity equals to that of the conventional Hodgkin–Huxley membrane at the same resting potential. The dendritic membrane has passive extra-synaptic conductivity $G_{p,d} = 0.0677 \, \text{mS cm}^{-2}$ and voltage-dependent synaptic conductivity of NMDA-type, G_{NMDA} associated with the reversal potentials $E_p = -65 \, \text{mV}$ and $E_{NMDA} = 0 \, \text{mV}$, respectively. Tonic activation of distributed (spatially homogeneous) NMDA inputs is simulated by introducing a uniform maximum value of NMDA conductivity $\overline{G}_{NMDA}$, so that the actual value of NMDA conductivity G_{NMDA} depends on the transmembrane potential E via the activating kinetic variable p: $G_{NMDA} = \overline{G}_{NMDA} \cdot p$.

Equation $dp/dt = \alpha_p(1 - p) - \beta_p p$ describes kinetics of a depolarization recovery of the NMDA channels from the extracellular magnesium block with the same rate constants α_p and β_p as those reported by Brodin *et al.* (1991). The specific membrane capacitance $C_m = 1 \, \mu\text{F cm}^{-2}$ and the cytoplasm resistivity $R_i = 100 \, \Omega \cdot \text{cm}$ are homogeneous throughout the cell.

The electrical structure of this path is characterized by the steady path profiles of the same set of physical values as those used in the previous examples. They are all taken after relaxation of the transients induced by the onset of tonic synaptic activation. These values are: the transmembrane potential $E(x)$; the partial and the total membrane conductivities $G_k(x)$ and $G_m(x) = \Sigma_k G_k(x)$; the effective reversal potential of the total membrane current $E_q(x) = \Sigma_k(G_k(x)/G_m(x))E_k(x)$; the total surface (per unit membrane area) and longitudinal (per unit path length) membrane current densities $J_m(x) = G_m(x)U(x)$ and $i(x) = \pi D J_m(x)$, where

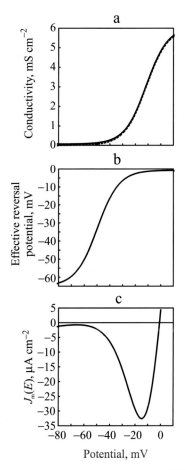

Figure 7.8 Steady-state local characteristics of the dendritic membrane as a function of the transmembrane potential E mV. a: Total membrane conductivity G_m and its synaptic G_{NMDA} component (solid and dashed lines, respectively), mS cm^{-2}; b: effective reversal potential E_q mV for the total transmembrane current; c: total surface current density (per unit membrane area), J_m μA cm^{-2}. (From Korogod and Kulagina, 1998a.)

$U(x) = E(x) - E_q(x)$ is the driving potential, D is the diameter, $G_k = G_{p,s}, G_{p,d}$ or G_{NMDA}, and $E_k = E_p$ or E_{NMDA}.

The function $-i(x) = \partial i_{core}(x)/\partial x$ linked with the increment of the core current per unit path length is used here for estimating the contribution of any element ∂x of the dendritic path to the total core current reaching the soma (Korogod and Kulagina, 1998b) (see Chapter 6). Local membrane properties of the dendrite are illustrated by the voltage dependence of the NMDA conductivity and its proportion of the total membrane conductivity (Figure 7.8, a). In a steady state, the effective reversal potential is a sigmoid function and the *I–V* plot is an N-shaped function of

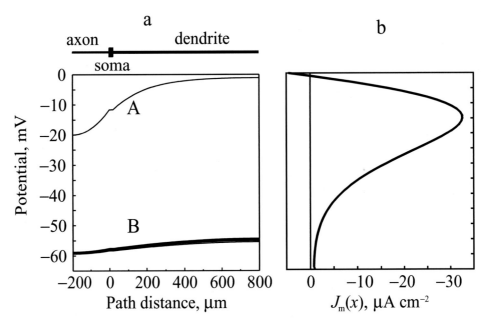

Figure 7.9 a: Path profiles of the steady-state transmembrane potential produced by tonic activation of NMDA-gated excitatory synaptic inputs homogeneously distributed along a passive dendrite. A: At a super-critical intensity $\overline{G}_{NMDA} = 6.10$ mS cm^{-2}; B: at ten subcritical intensities $\overline{G}_{NMDA}$ from 6.00 to 6.09 mS cm^{-2} separated by a small increment $\Delta\overline{G}_{NMDA} = 0.01$ mS cm^{-2}. The structure of the simulated neuron is shown above. Abscissae: distance from soma, μm; ordinates: potential, mV. b: Abscissae: surface current density, μA cm^{-2}; ordinates: potential, mV. (From Korogod and Kulagina, 1998a.)

the transmembrane potential (b and c, respectively). This N-shaped local characteristic has a negative slope within a voltage range from -66 to -15 mV, indicating the possibility of two depolarization steady states (Gutman, 1991) at a high (close to 0 mV) and a low level (close to the resting potential).

Introducing the homogeneous excitatory synaptic conductivity $\overline{G}_{NMDA}$ causes inhomogeneous depolarization, which is highest in the distal part and decays towards the soma and further to the distal end of the axon (Figure 7.9). Qualitatively, this behaviour looks like that observed in a path with a local steady I–V relation which has a positive slope over the whole range of membrane voltages. The steady depolarization is relatively small and slightly increases with each small increment $\Delta\overline{G}_{NMDA} = 0.01$ mS cm^{-2}, while the values of $\overline{G}_{NMDA}$ remain below a certain critical value (B). When a super-critical value ($\overline{G}_{NMDA} = 6.10$ mS cm^{-2}, in our example) is reached with the same small increment, a rather large increase in depolarization appears which reaches a very high level (A). A further increase in

$\overline{G}_{\text{NMDA}}$ produces an almost homogeneous depolarization in the most distal region of the path.

The path profiles obtained at subcritical and super-critical values of $\overline{G}_{\text{NMDA}}$ separated by small increments are shown in Figure 7.10, A–D and E–H, respectively. They correspond to one of the two stable states: the state of low depolarization close to the resting potential, which we call the *downstate*, and the state of high depolarization, close to the reversal potential of the excitatory synaptic current, the *upstate*.

In the downstate, the synaptic conductivity $G_{\text{NMDA}}(x)$ and the total conductivity $G_{\text{m}}(x)$ of the dendritic membrane are spatially inhomogeneous with the biggest values at the most depolarized dendritic tip (B). The driving potential $U(x) = E(x) - E_{\text{q}}(x)$ and the surface current density (per unit membrane area; A and C, respectively) increase with path distance from the soma. The core current increment per unit path length (D) reaches its greatest value ($0.2 \text{ pA } \mu\text{m}^{-1}$) at the distal dendritic end. Thus, in the downstate, the most depolarized distal dendritic sites supply more current to the soma than the proximal sites. This makes significant difference compared to dendrites having an *I–V* relation with positive slope.

In the upstate, with high dendritic depolarization, the synaptic conductivity G_{NMDA} is about one order of magnitude greater than that in the downstate and composes an overwhelming proportion of the total dendritic conductivity (Figure 7.10, F). The effective equilibrium potential approaches nearly the homogeneous partial equilibrium potential of the NMDA current (E, dashed line). The path profile of the driving potential is almost completely defined by the path profile of the transmembrane potential. The driving potential is nearly zero at the distal tip and reaches maximum negativity at the proximal end of the dendrite. The total membrane current is negative (inward) over the whole dendritic length. Its surface density is the greatest at the proximal end and decays towards the distal end of the dendrite (G). The contribution to the somatopetal core current is the biggest from the most proximal dendritic sites and rapidly decreases with increasing path distance from the soma (H). At the distal dendritic end, it is lower than in the downstate (0.15 and $0.2 \text{ pA } \mu\text{m}^{-1}$, respectively).

A further increase in the range of super-critical intensity of tonic activation leads to saturation of the membrane potential in the distal part of the dendrite. In this region, the transmembrane potential becomes homogeneous and equal to the effective equilibrium potential close to E_{NMDA}, and the current density is zero. The proximal border of such a zero-effective region approaches the soma as the intensity of tonic input increases further. In both downstate and upstate, the effective equilibrium potential remains at the initial level -65 mV in the axo-somatic part (A, E, dashed lines). Correspondingly, the driving potential and the current density per unit area are positive and decrease from their maxima at the soma towards the

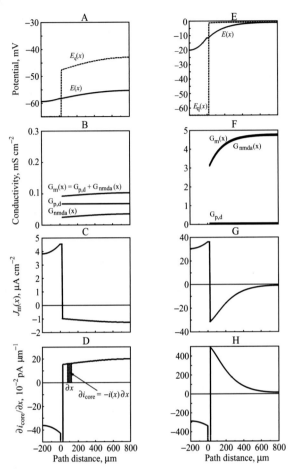

Figure 7.10 Path profiles of the electrical parameters of a passive dendrite under conditions of tonic activation of the voltage-dependent excitatory synaptic NMDA conductivities. Abscissae: Distance from soma, μm. Ordinates: Transmembrane E and effective reversal E_q potentials, mV (A, E); total membrane conductivity G_m and its synaptic G_{NMDA} and extra-synaptic $G_{p,d}$ components, mS cm^{-2} (B, F); surface density of total current (per unit membrane area) J_m, μA cm^{-2} (C, G); core current increment per unit path length $\partial i_{core}/\partial x$, pA μm^{-1} (D, H). Fragments A–D and E–H were obtained at sub- and super-critical synaptic intensities ($\overline{G}_{NMDA} = 6.0$ and 6.1 mS cm^{-2}, respectively). Dotted lines in D and H are eliminated peaks of the current density at the soma (-3.21 and -26.6 pA μm^{-1}). Striped area in D shows the contribution to the core current from the element ∂x. (From Korogod and Kulagina, 1998a.)

distal axon end. Since the soma has a much greater diameter than other parts of the neuron, there is a prominent peak of the outward current per unit length (D and H).

In this chapter, we have demonstrated how the electrical relations between dendritic sites along a single path determine the current delivered to the soma. We have explained which proximal or distal sites contribute more or less effectively to this somatopetal current and why. We have characterized the contributions by different estimates, depending on the dendritic membrane properties (passive or active) and the types of synaptic inputs (single-site or multiple and distributed). The charge transfer effectiveness is a good estimate in the case of passive dendrites activated at a single site and at a given moment in time. But only the universal estimate is relevant for cases of passive or active dendrites with distributed inputs (Korogod and Kulagina, 1998b).

Some conclusive facts can be drawn from the path profiles describing the spatial electrical relations:

(1) The type of local *I–V* relation of the dendritic membrane determines the type of proximal-to-distal relations along the dendritic path. The dendritic geometry controls these relations.

(2) As the dendritic path originates from a thick soma and ends with a thin tip, the structural asymmetry provokes an electrical asymmetry: a leaky origin and an almost sealed end involve a greater somatopetal and smaller somatofugal input conductance at each site. Thus, the inward input current at any site divides into unequal core currents with greater somatopetal and smaller somatofugal branches. Since the voltage drops in the direction of the net current flow, distal sites are more depolarized than proximal sites. The contribution to the core current at any site (the site effectiveness) can be found therefore from the local *I–V* relation and the membrane voltage.

(3) In dendrites with linear or non-linear *I–V* relations with positive slopes over the whole range of the membrane voltage, proximal sites are more effective than distal ones, whatever the synaptic inputs, single or distributed. The shorter the path, the greater the effectiveness because of the proximity of the sealed tip returning the current back into the dendrite.

(4) In dendrites with N-shaped *I–V* relations with positive and negative slopes, the proximal-to-distal relations depend on the specific range of the heterogeneous voltages along the path. If the membrane voltage is in the range of positive slope, the proximal-to-distal relations are similar to those described in (3); if it is in the range of negative slope, the relations are opposite: more depolarized distal sites generate greater inward currents and contribute more effectively to the somatopetal current. In cases in which different parts of the path are in ranges of different slopes, the relations are much more complex. For a given sign of the slope of the *I–V* relation, the slope steepness decides how large the difference in the transfer effectiveness between proximal and distal sites is. The steeper the slope, the larger the difference.

References

Abbot, L. F. (1991). Realistic synaptic inputs for model neural network. *Network*, **2**:245–258.

Barrett, J. N. and Crill, W. E. (1974). Influence of dendritic location and membrane properties on the effectiveness of synapses on cat motoneurons. *J. Physiol.*, **239**:325–345.

Bernander, O., Koch, C. and Douglas, R. J. (1994). Amplification and linearization of distal synaptic input to cortical pyramidal cells. *J. Neurophysiol.*, **72**:2743–2753.

Brodin, L., Tråvén, H. G. C., Lansner, A., Wallén, P., Ekeberg, O. E. and Grillner, S. (1991). Computer simulations of N-methyl-D-aspartate receptor-induced membrane properties in a neuron model. *J. Neurophysiol.*, **66**:473–484.

Carnevale, N. T., Tsai, K. Y., Clairborne, B. J. and Brown, T. H. (1997). Comparative electrotonic analysis of three classes of rat hippocampal neurons. *J. Neurophysiol.*, **78**:703–720.

Clements, J. D. and Redman, S. J. (1989). Cable properties of cat spinal motoneurones measured by combining voltage clamp, current clamp and intracellular staining. *J. Physiol.*, **409**:63–87.

Gutman, A. M. (1991). Bistability of dendrites. *J. Neural Syst.*, **1**:291–304.

Holmes, W. R. and Woody, C. D. (1989). Effects of uniform and non-uniform synaptic 'activation-distribution' on the cable properties of modeled cortical pyramidal neurons. *Brain Res.*, **505**:12–22.

Katz, B. and Miledi, R. (1963). A study of spontaneous miniature potentials in spinal motoneurones. *J. Physiol.*, **168**:389–422.

Koch, C. (1999). *Biophysics of Computation: Information Processing in Single Neurons*, New York, Oxford: Oxford University Press.

Korogod, S. M. (1996). Electro-geometrical coupling in non-uniform branching dendrites. Consequences for relative synaptic effectiveness. *Biol. Cybern.*, **74**:85–93.

Korogod, S. M. and Kulagina, I. B. (1998a). Conditions of dominant effectiveness of distal sites of active uniform dendrites with distributed tonic inputs. *Neurophysiology*, **30**(4/5):376–382.

Korogod, S. M. and Kulagina, I. B. (1998b). Geometry-induced features of current transfer in neuronal dendrites with tonically activated conductance. *Biol. Cybern.*, **79**:231–240.

Powers, R. K. and Binder, M. D. (1995). Effective synaptic current and motoneuron firing rate modulation. *J. Neurophysiol.*, **74**:793–801.

Powers, R. K., Robinson, F. R., Konodi, M. A. and Binder, M. D. (1992). Effective synaptic current can be estimated from measurements of neuronal discharges. *J. Neurophysiol.*, **68**:964–968.

Rospars, J.-P., Lansky, P., Tuckwel, H. C. and Vermeule, A. (1996). Coding of odor intensity in a steady-state deterministic model of an olfactory receptor neuron. *J. Comput. Neurosci.*, **3**:51–72.

Rusakov, D. A., Stewart, M. G. and Korogod, S. M. (1996). Branching of active dendritic spines as a mechanism for controlling synaptic efficacy. *Neuroscience*, **75**:315–323.

Schwindt, P. C. and Crill, W. E. (1980). Properties of a persistent inward current in normal and TEA-injected motoneurons. *J. Neurophysiol.*, **43**:1700–1724.

Stuart, G., Spruston, N. and Häusser (eds.) (2001). *Dendrites*, London: Oxford University Press.

8

Electrical structure of a bifurcation

After the single dendritic path analyzed in the preceding chapter, an elementary bifurcation introduces the simplest case of a second *discrete dimension* for navigating over the dendrites. A set of elementary bifurcations forms the so-called *binary tree*, which is most typical for dendritic arborizations of neurons. Obviously, the *bifurcation*, also named *binary branching* or *dichotomic branching* is topologically symmetrical but most often metrically asymmetrical, due to differences in lengths and/or diameters of the sister branches.

In this chapter, we study the proximal-to-distal electrical relationship in two sister paths by comparing sites situated at the same path distance from their common origin but on different paths. The path length of the shorter branch determines the path distance extent of the domain in which we can compare equidistant sites, since it is obvious that the most distal sites on the longer branch do not have equidistant counterparts on the shorter one! Remaining at the same path distance from the origin in the first continuous dimension and 'jumping' from one branch to the other in the second discrete dimension, we can compare electrical states of equidistant sites (Figure 8.1). Such a structure is most convenient for studying the impact of the metrical asymmetry of branching on the electrical structure of the paths. The difference in the electrical states reveals the critical impact of metrical asymmetry.

8.1 Theory for different configurations

Consider a simple example of metrical asymmetry: two branches of the same diameter d and different lengths, shorter l and longer $l' = l + \Delta l$ ($\Delta l > 0$) arising from the common origin. Assume that both branches have the same homogeneous electrical properties: the membrane and cytoplasm resistivity, R_m and R_i, respectively. This means equality of electrotonic length constant λ and characteristic semi-infinite cable input conductance G_∞. Compare the current transfer ratios at the sites situated at the same path distances x from the common origin point $x = 0$

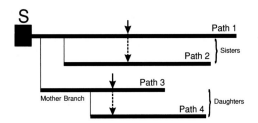

Figure 8.1 Schema of four dendritic paths (Path 1 to 4) with branching points at given distances from the soma (S).

but on different branches: $T(x)$ and $T'(x)$. For that consider the difference:

$$\Delta T(x) = T(x) - T'(x) \tag{8.1}$$

and relate this difference to the simplest metrical asymmetry indicator, the length difference in physical units Δl and dimensionless $\Delta L = \Delta l / \lambda$. The specific result depends on the boundary conditions posed at the distal ends of each branch, i.e. at $x = l$ of the shorter branch and $x = l'$ of the longer one. Consider the three conventional types of the boundary condition: (i) sealed-end, (ii) open-end (or voltage clamped to resting potential) and (iii) leaky-end with the leak conductance G_L.

8.1.1 Branches with sealed-ends

In a branch with 'sealed-end' boundary condition the current transfer ratio is defined by Equation (6.27). Correspondingly, the difference in $T(x)$ between each pair of equidistant sites located at $X = x/\lambda$ is:

$$\Delta T(X) = \frac{\cosh(L - X)}{\cosh(L)} - \frac{\cosh(L' - X)}{\cosh(L')} \tag{8.2}$$

Take this equation in the following form:

$$\Delta T(X) = \frac{\cosh(L - X)}{\cosh(L)} - \frac{\cosh(L + \Delta L - X)}{\cosh(L + \Delta L)} \tag{8.3}$$

Put the expansions:

$$\cosh(L - X) = \cosh(L)\cosh(X) - \sinh(L)\sinh(X) \tag{8.4}$$

and

$$\cosh(L + \Delta L - X) = \cosh(L + \Delta L)\cosh(X) - \sinh(L + \Delta L)\sinh(X) \tag{8.5}$$

into Equation (8.2), gather like terms, cancel opposite terms and employ the relation between hyperbolic functions. This gives:

$$\Delta T(X) = \sinh(X)[\tanh(L + \Delta L) - \tanh(L)] \tag{8.6}$$

This equation can be rewritten in terms of input conductances of the branches with sealed-ends, $G_{\text{inp}} = G_\infty \tanh(L)$ and $G'_{\text{inp}} = G_\infty \tanh(L + \Delta L)$:

$$\Delta T(X) = \sinh(X)(G'_{\text{inp}} - G_{\text{inp}})/G_\infty = \sinh(X)\Delta G_{\text{inp}}/G_\infty \tag{8.7}$$

8.1.2 Branches with open-ends

For the branches with 'open-end' boundary conditions, the current transfer ratio is defined by Equation (6.26). The corresponding equations defining the difference at equidistant sites $X = x/\lambda$ are as follows:

$$\Delta T(X) = \frac{\sinh(L - X)}{\sinh(L)} - \frac{\sinh(L' - X)}{\sinh(L')} \tag{8.8}$$

$$\Delta T(X) = \frac{\sinh(L - X)}{\sinh(L)} - \frac{\sinh(L + \Delta L - X)}{\sinh(L + \Delta L)} \tag{8.9}$$

$$\sinh(L - X) = \sinh(L)\cosh(X) - \cosh(L)\sinh(X) \tag{8.10}$$

$$\sinh(L + \Delta L - X) = \sinh(L + \Delta L)\cosh(X) - \cosh(L + \Delta L)\sinh(X) \tag{8.11}$$

$$\Delta T(X) = \sinh(X)[\coth(L + \Delta L) - \coth(L)] \tag{8.12}$$

Since multiplying $\coth(L + \Delta L)$ and $\coth(L)$ by the same value of the characteristic cable conductance G_∞ gives the input conductances of the branches $G_{\text{inp}} = G_\infty \coth(L)$ and $G'_{\text{inp}} = G_\infty \coth(L + \Delta L)$, that gives again Equation (8.7).

8.1.3 Branches with leaky-ends

For the branches with 'leaky-end' boundary conditions, the current transfer ratio is defined by Equation (6.29). The difference in the current transfer ratio between asymmetrical branches at equidistant sites is defined by more complicated equations given below. Consider two cases. In one case, the branches have different lengths (l and $l' > l$) and the same leak conductance (G_L) at their distal ends. In the other case, both branches have the same length (l), but the leak conductances at their ends are different (G_L and G'_L) that may correspond, for instance, to different continuations of the branches beyond a certain distance l.

Unequally long branches with the same leak

Denote the ratio of the leak and characteristic conductances entering in Equation (6.29) as follows

$$B = G_L/G_\infty \qquad (8.13)$$

In this case the difference in the current transfer ratio is:

$$\Delta T(X) = \frac{\cosh(L - X) + B\sinh(L - X)}{\cosh(L) + B\sinh(L)} - \frac{\cosh(L' - X) + B\sinh(L' - X)}{\cosh(L') + B\sinh(L')} \qquad (8.14)$$

This equation also can be reduced to the general form (Equation 8.7).
To prove that, first express Equation (8.14) in terms of the length increment:

$$\Delta T(X) = \frac{\cosh(L - X) + B\sinh(L - X)}{\cosh(L) + B\sinh(L)}$$
$$- \frac{\cosh(L + \Delta L - X) + B\sinh(L + \Delta L - X)}{\cosh(L + \Delta L) + B\sinh(L + \Delta L)} \qquad (8.15)$$

On the one hand, reducing the fractions to the same denomination and using the formulae for a hyperbolic sine and cosine sum of two arguments, $(L + \Delta L)$ or L and X, with further gathering of like terms and cancelling of opposite terms in Equation (8.15) leads to the following expression:

$$\Delta T(X) = \sinh(X)(1 - B^2)\frac{\tanh(L) - \tanh(L + \Delta L)}{[1 + B\tanh(L)][1 + B\tanh(L + \Delta L)]} \qquad (8.16)$$

On the other hand, from the difference of the input conductances of the two leaky cables with assigned properties:

$$\Delta G_{\text{inp}} = G_{\text{inp}} - G'_{\text{inp}} = G_\infty \left(\frac{\tanh(L) + B}{1 + B\tanh(L)} - \frac{\tanh(L + \Delta L) + B}{1 + B\tanh(L + \Delta L)} \right)$$

one gets:

$$\Delta G_{\text{inp}} = G_\infty(1 - B^2)\frac{\tanh(L) - \tanh(L + \Delta L)}{[1 + B\tanh(L)][1 + B\tanh(L + \Delta L)]} \qquad (8.17)$$

Equation (8.7) directly follows from Equations (8.16) and (8.17) and hence completes the proof.

Equally long branches with different leaks

In this case, because of the difference in the leak conductance, the ratio of the conductances used in further formulae are:

$$B = G_L/G_\infty \qquad \text{and} \qquad B' = G'_L/G_\infty \qquad (8.18)$$

With this notation the current transfer ratio is:

$$\Delta T(X) = \frac{\cosh(L-X) + B\sinh(L-X)}{\cosh(L) + B\sinh(L)} - \frac{\cosh(L-X) + B'\sinh(L-X)}{\cosh(L) + B'\sinh(L)}$$

(8.19)

Applying to Equation (8.19) the same operations as applied to Equation (8.15) one gets:

$$\Delta T(X) = \sinh(X)(B - B')\frac{1}{[\cosh(L) + B\sinh(L)][\cosh(L) + B'\sinh(L)]}$$

(8.20)

On the other hand, from the corresponding difference of input conductances:

$$\Delta G_{\text{inp}} = G_{\text{inp}} - G'_{\text{inp}} = G_{\infty}\left(\frac{\tanh(L) + B}{1 + B\tanh(L)} - \frac{\tanh(L) + B'}{1 + B'\tanh(L)}\right)$$

it follows:

$$\Delta G_{\text{inp}} = G_{\infty}(B - B')\frac{1}{[\cosh(L) + B\sinh(L)][\cosh(L) + B'\sinh(L)]} \quad (8.21)$$

From Equations (8.20) and (8.21) again one directly gets Equation (8.7).

Several narrative conclusions follow from the expression (8.7) describing the difference in the current transfer ratio between equidistant sites on asymmetrical branches in general form. Whatever the boundary conditions at the distal ends are, the difference $\Delta T(x)$ is determined by the same four factors: (i) the common 'spatial' factor $\sinh(X)$ depending on the electrotonic path distance $X = x/\lambda$ from the common origin; (ii) the characteristic input conductance of the semi-infinite dendritic cable G_{∞}; (iii) and (iv), respectively, the input conductances G_{inp} and G'_{inp} of the branches as seen from their common origin. The hyperbolic sine $\sinh(X)$ is a positive increasing function of the path distance. This means that the difference in $T(X)$ between equidistant sites always increases with the path distance. Correspondingly, the path profiles $T(x)$ and $T'(X)$ diverge along asymmetrical paths. The difference is the greatest at the path distance x equal to the length of the shorter branch l.

How big is this divergence? Other factors must be considered to find out the response. At a given path distance x, the difference $\Delta T(X)$ is directly proportional to the difference in the input conductances between the sister branches, $\Delta G_{\text{inp}} = G_{\text{inp}} - G'_{\text{inp}}$. The input conductances are positive increasing functions of the path length and hence the metrical asymmetry directly determines this factor. Inverse proportional dependence of $\Delta T(X)$ on the characteristic input conductance $G_{\infty} = $

$(\pi/2)(d)^{3/2}(R_m R_i)^{-1/2}$ indicates how the branch diameter and electrical parameters are involved.

In the next section, we use specific examples, typical of dendritic arborizations, to illustrate the general notions just described. We replace the model of the single path by the binary branching dendrite composed of a parent branch giving rise to two daughter branches, symmetrical in one case and asymmetrical in the other (see Figure 8.1). As in the preceding chapter, we use the same model of the neuron (Figure 7.2) with passive or active membrane properties and the same protocols of simulation.

8.2 Electrical structure of passive branching paths with single-site inputs

For a given diameter of the parent branch, $d_0 = 5\,\mu$m, the diameters of the daughter branches ($d_1 = d_2 = 5\,\mu$m, $3.1498\,\mu$m and $1.9844\,\mu$m) are chosen so that the geometrical ratios $GR = (d_1^{3/2} + d_2^{3/2})/d_0^{3/2}$ representing deviation from '3/2 power' law for the equivalent cylinder (Rall, 1989) are equal to 2, 1 and 0.5. The dendrites with these geometries are electrotonically similar to single un-branched dendrites with step-wise increased, unchanged and step-wise decreased diameters (Clements and Redman, 1989). Relationships between voltage gradients in pre- and post-node points are more complicated than those between pre- and post-step changes in diameter. An important difference is that the post-node core current entering any daughter branch is only a proportion of the pre-node core current, partitioned according to the input conductances of the sister branches.

Dendritic path profiles of voltage generated by a steady current applied to the soma are illustrated for cases of symmetrical and asymmetrical branching with open and sealed ends in Figures 8.2 and 8.3 respectively. In both figures, cases of symmetrical branches are represented by the dashed lines and the asymmetrical cases by the solid lines. Figure 8.2 illustrates the computed voltage profiles for the open-end condition. Figure 8.3 illustrates the computed voltage profiles for the sealed-end condition.

8.2.1 Somatofugal voltage along branching paths

Symmetrical branching

In the case of symmetrical branching, the ratios of the input conductances are $G_{1in}/G_{2in} = 1$ and $G_{1in}/(G_{1in} + G_{2in}) = 0.5$, the daughter voltage profiles are identical and the ratio of the post-node voltage gradients is $\Psi_{12} = \mathcal{E}_1/\mathcal{E}_2 = 1$ (Equation 6.38). The trans-node behaviour of the gradient (Figure 8.2) is mainly determined by the ratio of the pre- to post-node diameters. When these diameters are

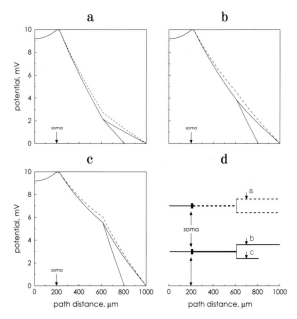

Figure 8.2 Somatofugal voltage distribution along open-end symmetrical (dashed lines) and asymmetrical (continuous lines) branching dendrites (d) with three different relationships of pre- and post-node diameters specified in the text. (From Korogod, 1996.)

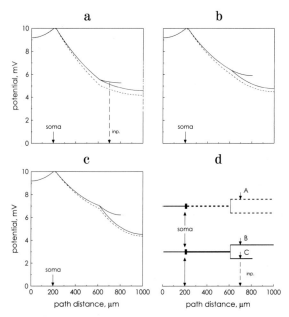

Figure 8.3 Same as Figure 8.2 but with sealed-end conditions. Arrows A–C indicate sites of injection of the same testing current to estimate the somatopetal charge transfer effectiveness. (From Korogod, 1996.)

equal, then at the node there is a twofold somatofugal decrease in the gradient (a): $\Psi_{10} = \mathcal{E}_1/\mathcal{E}_0 = 0.5$ (Equation 6.39).

This behaviour is similar to that occurring at the site of the step increase in diameter of the un-branched dendrite (Figure 7.3). The thinner the daughter branches are, the smaller the pre-node gradient. It becomes equal to or less than the post-node one in both boundary conditions.

Asymmetrical branching

In the case of asymmetry, the pre- and post-node gradients relationship is governed by the same factors as above, although both gradients are less than their symmetrical counterparts under sealed-end conditions, and vice versa under open-end conditions. The ratios between the post-node gradients in the unequally long sister branches are reciprocal under sealed-end and open-end boundary conditions. With equality of the diameters, the ratio of the post-node gradients is determined by the ratio of the branch input conductances (Equation 6.38). The shorter branch has a smaller input conductance and post-node gradient than the longer one under sealed-end conditions, and vice versa under open-end conditions. Thus, metrical asymmetry induces a perturbation in the voltage gradient that leads to divergence of the post-nodal voltage path profiles.

8.2.2 Somatopetal charge transfer along branching paths

We apply the same simulation protocol to the symmetrical or asymmetrical bifurcating dendrite as for the non-branching dendrites described in the previous chapter. The evaluations of the current transfer effectiveness (transfer ratio) T_{d0} are obtained in two ways. First, by calculating Equation (6.24), that is the steady somatofugal voltage profiles, as shown in Figure 8.3, a. Second, by calculating the ratio of voltage-time integrals of the somatic EPSPs produced by the same transient synaptic currents injected at the dendritic site under study and at the soma (Figure 8.4).

In this example, the relative effectiveness of symmetrical sister branches is equally low and the shorter branch is more effective among asymmetrical ones. In each case, both values of T obtained in the two different ways are practically identical.

8.3 Electrical structure of a bifurcation receiving distributed tonic inputs

We apply the same simulation protocol to the bifurcating symmetrical or asymmetrical dendrite as for non-branching dendrites described in the previous chapter (see Figure 7.2). We keep the same membrane properties for computing the electrical

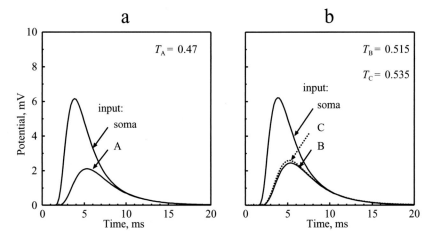

Figure 8.4 EPSPs at the soma in response to somatic and dendritic injections of transient synaptic current at sites indicated in Figure 8.3, a, d. Values of the relative effectiveness defined by voltage-time integrals are given at the right top corner. (From Korogod, 1996.)

profiles produced by tonic active inputs homogeneously distributed over the dendrites. The simulated neuron has the same cylinder-shaped soma (20 μm length, 22.5 μm diameter), an axon (200 μm length, 3 μm diameter) and a binary branching dendrite. The dendritic bifurcation is symmetrical or asymmetrical. The length and diameter of the mother branch is the same (380 μm and 5 μm, respectively). In the model with symmetrical bifurcation, both daughter branches have the same lengths as the mother branch. In the model with asymmetrical bifurcation, the daughter branches are 380 and 195 μm in length. With the given diameter of the mother branch ($d_0 = 5$ μm), equal diameters of the daughter branches are chosen ($d_1 = d_2 = 5$ μm, 3.1498 μm and 1.9844 μm) so that the geometrical ratios $GR = (d_1^{3/2} + d_2^{3/2})/d_0^{3/2}$ representing deviation from 3/2-power law for the equivalent passive cylinder are 2, 1 and 1/2 (Rall, 1989). The symmetrically passive branching dendrite with these geometries is reducible to electrotonically equivalent un-branching passive dendrites with stepwise increased and stepwise decreased uniform diameters at the site corresponding to the bifurcation node (Rall, 1959; Clements and Redman, 1989). GR expression in terms of 3/2 powers is used to facilitate comparison with the conventional analysis of complex dendrites.

Three figures are used to illustrate the results of the computations. In each case, the membrane potentials, the total membrane current density per unit area, the increment of the core current per unit path length and the somatopetal current transfer effectiveness from single sources are calculated as a function of the path distance from the soma. But each figure illustrates three different cases of diameter relationship between mother and both daughter branches. Figure 8.5 shows the

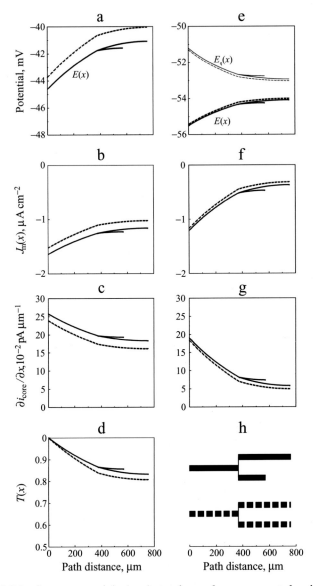

Figure 8.5 Membrane potentials (a, e), total membrane current density per unit area (b, f), increment of the core current per unit path length (c, g) and somatopetal current transfer effectiveness from single sources (d) (ordinates) as a function of path distance from the soma along symmetrical (dashed lines) and asymmetrical (solid lines) branches with passive (a–d) or active (e–g) extra-synaptic membranes resulting from steady uniform activation of excitatory conductivity. Diameters of mother and both daughter branches are equal ($d_0 = d_1 = d_2 = 5\,\mu m$) giving the geometrical ratio $GR = (d_1^{3/2} + d_2^{3/2})/d_0^{3/2} = 2$ such that two symmetrical daughter branches are electronically equivalent to extension of the mother branch by a uniform cylinder of increased diameter. (From Korogod and Kulagina, 1998.)

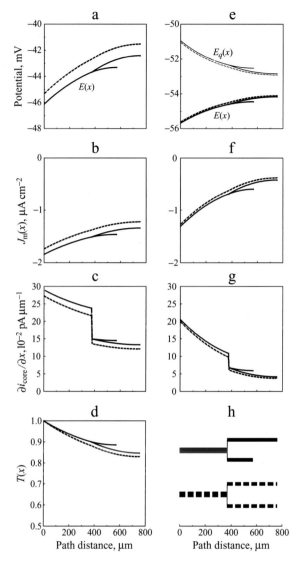

Figure 8.6 Same as Figure 8.5 but with $d_0 = 5\,\mu m$ and $d_1 = d_2 = 3.1498\,\mu m$ ($GR = 1$, symmetrical branching electrotonically equivalent to uniform cylinder of unchanged diameter d_0). (From Korogod and Kulagina, 1998.)

case in which the diameters of mother and daughter branches are equal. Figure 8.6 shows the case in which the diameter of the mother branch is larger than the two diameters of the daughter branches, which are equal and with a relation $GR = 1$. Finally, Figure 8.7 gives an example in which the diameter of the mother branch is also larger than the two diameters of the daughter branches, which are equal, but with a relation $GR = 0.5$. To facilitate comparison, we add the plots of the relative

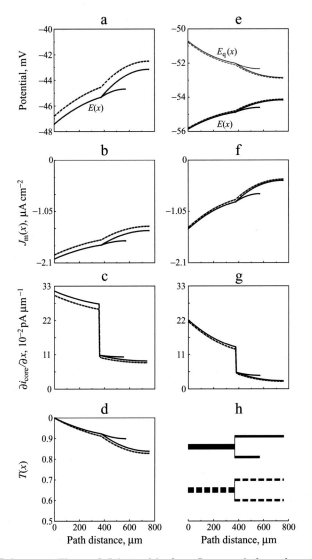

Figure 8.7 Same as Figure 8.5 but with $d_0 = 5\,\mu\text{m}$ and $d_1 = d_2 = 1.9844\,\mu\text{m}$ ($GR = 0.5$, symmetrical branching electrotonically equivalent to a uniform cylinder of unchanged diameter $d_0/2$). (From Korogod and Kulagina, 1998.)

effectiveness of the charge transfer from single-site sources $T(x)$ computed for the same structure in each figure.

8.3.1 Dendritic membrane **I–V** relation with positive slope

First, we consider a passive or active dendrite with Hodgkin–Huxley type conductances receiving distributed tonic activation (Figures 8.5 to 8.7, see above).

Its membrane is characterized by an I–V relation with positive slope. The distributed tonic synaptic action is simulated by introducing a constant homogeneous voltage-independent synaptic conductivity G_s (see Section 7.2.2).

Introducing a steady uniform excitatory conductance $G_s = 0.0677 \, \text{mS cm}^{-2}$ along branching dendrites leads to the generation of steady voltages and currents with inhomogeneous path profiles. The depolarization shift in the transmembrane potential $E(x)$ is spatially inhomogeneous and increases with the path distance from the soma (a and e in Figures 8.5 to 8.7). The slope of the path profile of the depolarization decreases with path distance from the soma, being positive in the dendrite. Both the level and the gradient of the depolarization are greater in the passive dendrite than in the active Hodgkin–Huxley type (a and e in Figures 8.5 to 8.7). The equilibrium potential $E_q(x)$ is shifted to depolarization and its path profiles are uniform $E_q = -32.5 \, \text{mV}$ in the passive dendrites and non-uniform and decreasing with path distance from the soma in the active dendrite (e, two upper profiles in Figures 8.5 to 8.7). Thus, the negative driving potential $E(x) - E_q(x)$ decreases with path distance from the soma and its value and the rate of somatofugal decrease are greater when the dendritic membrane is active. The total transmembrane current is negative and inward and its densities per unit area and per unit length decrease with increasing path distance from the soma in both passive and active dendrites (f, g in Figures 8.5 to 8.7). This leads to a corresponding somatopetal increase in the core current increment, that is the elementary contribution $\partial i_{\text{core}} = -i(x)\partial x$ to the net current reaching the soma. The current collected from the branching dendrite is consumed in the axo-somatic part with the peak at the soma (not shown).

The path profiles of the potentials and currents in the branching dendrites have features that are induced by their specific branching geometry. The symmetrical daughter branches are identical in the path distributions of the conductances, voltages, currents and relative charge transfer effectiveness (overlapping dashed lines in Figures 8.5 to 8.7). At the branching node, the gradient of the potential is discontinuous whereas the potential is continuous. When passing the node in the somatofugal direction, the slope of the path profile of the dendritic depolarization abruptly decreases or increases if the geometrical ratio GR is 2 or $1/2$, respectively. These values correspond to the electrotonically equivalent non-branching dendrite with a stepwise increase or decrease in diameter at the path distance equal to the length of the mother branch. In a symmetrically branching passive dendrite with $GR = 1$, there is still a trans-node break in the voltage gradient, so that the slope is slightly greater on the daughter-branch side than on the mother-branch side of the node. However, the voltage gradient is continuous if the diameters of the daughter branches are $d_1 = d_2 = 3.55 \, \mu\text{m}$, corresponding to $(d_1^{1/2} + d_2^{1/2})/d_0^{1/2} = 1$.

In the same dendrites with passive membrane properties computed for reference, the relative effectiveness $T(x)$ of the somatopetal charge transfer from single-site sources is a continuous decaying function of path distance from the soma (d in Figures 8.5 to 8.7). The slope of its somatofugal decay is continuous along uniform branches, but discontinuous at the branching node with the same GR-dependent trans-node behaviour as that of the voltage gradient (see also the above section). Namely, for $GR = 1$ and $1/2$, the post-node slope is greater, and for $GR = 2$ less than the pre-node slope. The slope is continuous at the branching point (i.e. pre- and post-node values are equal) only in the case of symmetrical branching with $d_1 = d_2 = 3.55\,\mu\text{m}$ corresponding to $(d_1^2 + d_2^2)/d_0^2 = 1$ (not shown).

In the case of asymmetrical branching, the path profiles of all electrical values along sister branches diverge. Comparison of somatofugally equidistant sites of these two branches (Figures 8.5 to 8.7) shows that the sites of the shorter branch have: (i) smaller transmembrane depolarization; (ii) greater depolarization shift of the effective equilibrium potential $E_q(x)$ from the initial resting value -65 mV in the case of the active dendrite; (iii) consequently, a greater driving potential $E(x) - E_q(x)$ of the total transmembrane current; (iv) a greater surface density of the transmembrane current; (v) a greater elementary contribution to the somatopetal core current and finally (vi) a greater relative effectiveness of the somatopetal charge transfer from single-site sources $T(x)$.

The voltage $E(x)$ and most of the voltage-dependent membrane characteristics such as the total conductivity and current density per unit area $G_m(x)$ and $J_m(x)$ and the effective equilibrium potential $E_q(x)$ are always continuous at the bifurcation. However, the profiles of the path increment of the core current $\partial i_{\text{core}}/\partial x$ are generally discontinuous at the branching node. The continuity takes place only when the diameters of the mother and both daughter branches are equal (Figure 8.5, c, g). Otherwise, these characteristics abruptly decrease when passing the node from a thicker mother branch to a thinner daughter branch (c, g in Figures 8.6 and 8.7) or increase when the pre-node and post-node diameters are in the inverse relation. A greater difference between the pre- and post-node values of $\partial i_{\text{core}}/\partial x = -i(x)$ corresponds to a greater trans-node change in diameter. For the same geometry of branching, this difference is greater in the passive dendrite than in the active Hodgkin–Huxley type.

8.3.2 Dendritic membrane with N-shaped I–V relation

Now, we consider the electrical structure of the bifurcating dendrite with N-shaped I–V relation provided by a minimum sufficient cocktail of conductances including voltage-dependent non-inactivating synaptic conductance of NMDA-type. The geometry of the model is the same as one of the above considered examples

(Figure 8.5). Namely, the diameters of mother and both daughter branches were equal $d_0 = d_1 = d_2 = 5\,\mu m$ giving the geometrical ratio $GR = (d_1^{3/2} + d_2^{3/2})/d_0^{3/2} = 2$. The membrane properties and simulation protocols are the same as in the previous chapter (Section 7.2.4).

Introducing a homogeneous maximum synaptic conductance $\overline{G}_{NMDA}$, which corresponds to a certain level of tonic activation of the dendritic excitatory synaptic inputs, causes spatially inhomogeneous depolarization of the membrane potential. The level of the depolarization depends on the intensity of the activation (Figure 7.10).

The bifurcating dendrite becomes electrically bistable with the typical downstate and upstate (Figure 8.8, A–D and E–H, respectively). The values of $\overline{G}_{NMDA}$ sub-critical and super-critical for the bistability of this bifurcating dendrite are $5.3\,mS\,cm^{-2}$ and $5.4\,mS\,cm^{-2}$, respectively (they are lower than those for the non-branching dendrites considered above). The membrane depolarization (Figure 8.8, A, E) in both states is the greatest at the distal ends of the branching dendrite and decreases towards the soma. In the asymmetrical bifurcation, the longer sister branch is more depolarized than the shorter one. Along the whole dendrite the low-level (downstate) depolarization is within the range of the negative slope of the local $I–V$ relation. The high-level (upstate) depolarization is outside the range of the negative slope and is in the range of the positive slope.

The impact of asymmetry on the current transfer along the branching dendrite is elucidated by analyzing path profiles of other parameters of the dendritic membrane in the downstate and upstate (Figure 8.8, A–D and E–H). With transition between the downstate and the upstate, changes occur in the voltage-dependent membrane conductance (B and F), in the effective reversal potential of the total transmembrane current (dashed lines in A and E), in the density of the total transmembrane current per unit membrane area (C and G) and in the increment of the core current per unit length of the dendritic path (D and H). In the dendrite, the total membrane current is negative (inward) while it is positive (outward) in the axo-somatic part.

It is a critical feature of the profiles that, in each branch, the distal sites have the total membrane current density and the effectiveness of the somatopetal transfer of the core current greater or smaller than the proximal sites in the downstate or the upstate. Even more important is that the relation between the longer and the shorter daughter branches in both the total membrane current density and the effectiveness of the somatopetal current transfer become inverse after transition of the dendritic depolarization from downstate to upstate. As compared with the shorter branch, the equidistant sites of the longer branch are more effective in the downstate and less effective in the upstate of depolarization.

In bifurcations with other combinations of diameters of the mother and daughter branches, the relationships between electrical profiles along asymmetrical sister

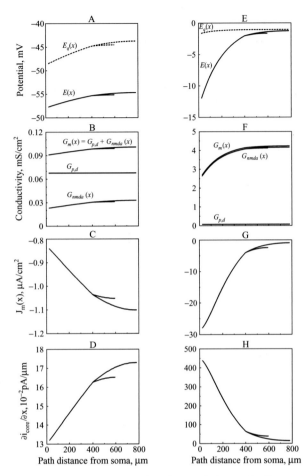

Figure 8.8 Electrical parameters as functions of the path distance x from the soma (abscissae) along branching electrically bistable dendrite with tonically activated voltage-dependent excitatory synaptic conductance (NMDA-type). A, E: The transmembrane potential $E(x)$ (solid lines) and effective equilibrium potential of the total transmembrane current $E_q(x)$ (dashed lines). B, F: The total membrane conductivity G_m with its synaptic G_{NMDA} and passive extra-synaptic $G_{p,d}$ components. C, G: The total current per unit membrane area J_m. D, H: The core current increment per unit path length $\partial i_{core}/\partial x$. A–D and E–H were obtained at sub- and super-critical synaptic intensity ($\overline{G}_{NMDA} = 5.3$ and $5.4\,\text{mS cm}^{-2}$), respectively. (From Kulagina, 1998.)

branches are qualitatively similar to those described above. The main difference is more or less prominent discontinuity of the core current profiles observed at the branching node with 'mismatched' cross-sectional areas of the adjacent branches, the effect resembling those found in bifurcations with positively sloped I–V relations (see previous subsection).

8.4 Recapitulation and conclusions

Several conclusions can be drawn from our computations:

(1) Any bifurcation is topologically symmetrical, but is metrically either symmetrical or asymmetrical depending on the equality or inequality of the sister branch lengths and/or diameters.

(2) The transfer properties of equidistant sites on the sister paths depend on the 'proximal-to-distal' relations along the path and are determined by metrical parameters: the path length and diameter. The equidistant sites are similar or dissimilar.

(3) Metrically symmetrical sister paths of equal lengths and diameters are identical in their transfer properties, provided that the local $I-V$ relation of the dendritic membrane and the synaptic inputs are the same. The reason for that is the identity of each pair of equidistant sites along the sister paths. This identity is represented graphically by the overlapped sister path profiles of electrical parameters, i.e. membrane voltages or currents. The sister profiles are indistinguishable and, in that sense, are called 'degenerative.'

(4) Metrical asymmetry induces the difference between equidistant sites in their transfer properties and thereby in electrical states. The greater the metrical asymmetry is, the greater the electrical difference between the sister paths. In this case, the sister path profiles diverge. In other words, breaking the metrical symmetry of the bifurcation removes the degeneracy of electrical profiles of the sister paths.

(5) The specific 'path-to-path' relation is determined by the difference in the 'proximal-to-distal' relation along the sister paths and thus depends both on the type of local $I-V$ relation of the dendritic membrane and on the type of synaptic input. The 'proximal-to-distal' relation of any type is exalted along the shorter branch compared to the longer sister branch.

(6) In a bifurcation with homogeneous membrane properties and any type of synaptic input (single-site or distributed), the sites along the shorter branch contribute to the somatopetal core current more efficiently than equidistant sites on the longer branch, whatever the local $I-V$ relation. There is one exception. This special case is a bifurcation with an N-shaped (type 3) local $I-V$ relation in the electrical downstate when the dendritic depolarization is within the range of the negative slope of the $I-V$ curve. Here, the sites along the shorter branch are less effective than those along the longer one.

(7) The heterogeneous diameter (d) modulates the effectiveness of the sister branches. Thinner branches are less effective. It is so because the local transmembrane leak conductance and the core conductance are proportional to different powers of the diameter: d^1 and d^2, respectively. In passive bifurcation with single-site inputs at each site along the thinner branch, the proportion between the core current and membrane leak current is changed in favour of the leak (decreased effectiveness) in proportion to a decreased d. In the dendrites with distributed synaptic inputs, the contribution to the core current in the thinner branch is smaller because of reduced membrane surface

area: given a surface current density, the intensity of the transmembrane current is proportional to the diameter (perimeter πd).

References

Clements, J. D. and Redman, S. J. (1989). Cable properties of cat spinal motoneurones measured by combining voltage clamp, current clamp and intracellular staining. *J. Physiol.*, **409**:63–87.

Korogod, S. M. (1996). Electro-geometrical coupling in non-uniform branching dendrites. Consequences for relative synaptic effectiveness. *Biol. Cybern.*, **74**:85–93.

Korogod, S. M. and Kulagina, I. B. (1998). Geometry-induced features of current transfer in neuronal dendrites with tonically activated conductance. *Biol. Cybern.*, **79**:231–240.

Kulagina, I. B. (1998). Transfer properties of branching dendrites with tonically activated inputs. *Neurophysiology*, **30**:316–319.

Rall, W. (1959). Branching dendritic trees and motoneurons membrane resistivity. *Exp. Neurol.*, **1**:491–527.

Rall, W. (1989). Cable theory for dendritic neurons. In Koch, C. and Segev, I. (eds.), *Methods in Neuronal Modeling*, p. 9–62, Cambridge, Mass.: MIT Press.

9

Geography of the dendritic space

Biological neurons have complex and diverse *shape* and *size*, which are mainly defined by their dendritic arborization (see Chapter 2). Considering the complex arborizations given by nature one can recognize the elementary structures considered in Chapters 7 and 8. The uniform segments, symmetrical or, more often, asymmetrical bifurcations as structural components are present in biological arborizations en masse and in various, unpredictable combinations. The geometrical information required for building the electrical structure of biological dendrites is the same as for the elementary artificial dendritic structures: the branching pattern, lengths and diameters of the branches, whereas the 3D organization does not matter. In the 3D biological arborization, because of the complexity all these structural details are seen hardly if at all, and so retrieving and relating the structural and electrical features are hampered. To deal with this problem we have to separate different aspects of geometry of the dendritic space.

One aspect could be considered as intrinsic, irrelevant of the 3D arrangement of a neuron in the space of the brain or spinal cord. The components of the dendritic structure are characterized only in terms of their lengths and diameters. The multiplicity of the structural components (paths, branches and bifurcations) imparts the *complexity* to the biological dendrites. In a given arborization, one meets unpredictably connected branches with unpredictably varying lengths and heterogeneous diameters and, in that sense, the dendritic geometry is *stochastic* both *topologically* and *metrically*. Since the difference in length and diameter between dendritic branches and paths is a determinative indicator of metrical asymmetry, we name this aspect *the whole arborization metrical asymmetry*. This one-dimension (path distance) geometrical aspect is sufficient for computations of the electrical structure of the biological arborization. However, it is not sufficient for understanding how the synaptic inputs arriving from different sources in the 3D space of the population are processed by the dendrites embedded in this space. For that, another 3D (extrinsic) aspect of the dendritic geometry should be considered.

Indeed, the arborizations are *3D structures* embedded in the 3D space of the nervous tissue. In the 3D space, the dendritic branches plough unpredictably meandering ways of randomly varying direction that impart new dimensions to the (geo)metrical stochasticity of the arborization structure. One can choose planar polar, volume cylindrical or spherical coordinates for appropriate description of the arborization spatial structure. According to the coordinate dependence of its elements the structure can be symmetrical or asymmetrical in 3D. Collectively these structures define layered, laminar or nuclear organization of parts of the spinal cord and the brain. The arborization forms a special kind of complex stochastic space, the dendritic space. It is this space, in which non-electrical forces separate the charges and create the electric fields translocating the charges and producing electrical events considered as neuronal signals.

The dendritic space of each neuron is the bearer and determinant of its electrical transfer properties. In this chapter we consider how the bearers are structurally composed and then, in the following chapters we consider how the dendritic space determines its electrical properties. Navigation in this intricate space requires special maps, which have to represent clearly the spatial structure of the arborization. To describe the structure of the dendritic space one has, like in terrestrial geography, to distinguish characteristic elements of the 'dendritic landscape', to choose the reference landmarks (coordinate system) for defining mutual location of the elements, and even to perform spatial transformations for getting a clearer view of the inter-relation between the structural elements. We start with a description of the general 'geography' of the dendritic space, taking well-known neuron types as examples. Then we describe specific instances of the these types of neurons collected in the database of digitized cells that we use for simulation studies of the geometry-induced electrical features.

9.1 Dendritic arborization in 3D and 2D representations

Complex spatial objects require relevant tools for visualization of their structure and properties. Maps of different kinds serve as such tools. One can notice some analogy between dendritic map-making and celestial or terrestrial cartography: original 3D objects have to be transformed into other 3D or 2D objects for the sake of clarity of their structural details. For instance, map-makers first observe the Earth as a 3D object close to an oblate spheroid. It is then represented by a terrestrial global 3D sphere or by flat 2D maps obtained by corresponding transformation of the originally measured 3D spatial data. Several types of cartographical projections (cylindrical, azimuthal etc.) on 2D map planes have been invented for better visualization of the Earth landscape. The 3D globe and 2D maps are further used for visualization of properties of different geographical regions.

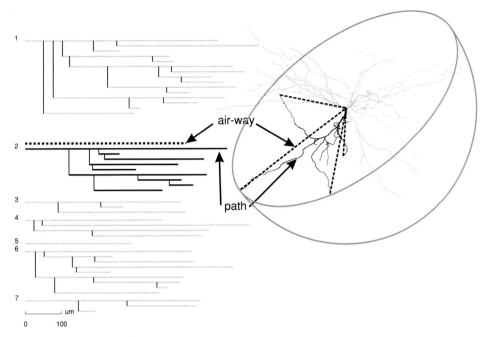

Figure 9.1 Arborization of seven dendrites of an abducens motoneuron in 2D dendrogram (left) and 3D (right) representations. Dendrite No. 2 is black and others are grey. Air-way extents are shown by dashed lines for four of the nine paths of this dendrite. For the longest path (indicated by arrows) the air-way extent is also shown by a dashed line near the corresponding dendrogram.

For instance, mapping the borders between countries gives a political map of the world. Putting colour-coded physical values such as temperature on the geographical maps provides a temperature map that improves understanding of the weather.

The dendritic arborization of the neuron is a peculiar 3D spatial object (e.g. Figure 9.1). It is visualized as an original 3D image projected onto certain projection plane(s) or as a transformed flat image called a *dendrogram* (see Chapter 2). The natural image of the arborization seen in the microscope is formed by meandering branching 3D curves of heterogeneous thickness (Figure 9.1). Computer-aided measurements of 3D coordinates and diameters of the curves provide digitized data for further spatial transformation and building the dendrograms (Figure 9.1), which can be considered as the kind of cartographical projections of the original 3D image. The two representations of the same arborization serve different purposes.

The world of the neuron with its dendrites is soma-centric. The peri-somatic volume is the 'meeting space' shared by the dendrites and the pre-synapic axons contacting them. The pattern of the dendritic branching in this volume determines the sampling (retrieving) of pre-synaptic signals from the 3D space. Describing the geography of the 3D dendritic space gives spatial reference points and guiding lines for specification of the spatial signal reception by the dendrites. For this world the cardinal directions and the compass rose are made of the *air-way* radii emanating from the conventional centre at the soma. A family of air-way radii drawn from the somatic origin to the tips or other characteristic sites of the paths of a given dendrite define the spatial angle as the *branching space* or *field* of the dendrite. These fields can be morphologically characterized in terms of their orientation, extent and shape in the 3D space, occupancy by (density of) dendritic branches etc. These characteristics are used for classification of the dendritic spatial patterns together with some functional assumptions (Ramón-Moliner and Nauta, 1966; Migliore and Shepherd, 2005).

For our restricted purposes applying an appropriate classification to distinct parts of the space occupied by the dendrites is based mainly on the spatial radiation of the dendrites in the peri-somatic space (Fiala and Harris, 1999). According to this classification, one can particularly distinguish dendritic fields with *laminar, spherical, cylindrical, conical, bi-conical and fan radiation* (see Table 1.2 in Fiala and Harris, 1999). In fact, such classifications and further subclassifications are based on the symmetry of distribution of dendritic branches in the 3D space. For instance, dendrites branching within a sphere centred at the soma are an example of spherical radiation, which can be symmetrical or asymmetrical. In the symmetrical case, the dendrites radiate in all directions from the cell body giving the *stellate*-type arborization characteristic of spinal motoneurons and other cells in the subcortical nuclei and cerebellum. If the dendrite radiates from the cell body in directions restricted to part of a sphere, the angular distribution of the dendrites is asymmetrical and the spherical radiation is of the *partial-type* characteristic of the neurons situated at the edges of so-called 'closed' nuclei (e.g. Clarke's column or vestibular nuclei). Examples of conical or bi-conical radiations are provided by the dendrites, which radiate within conical or paraboloidal regions oriented in one direction or in two opposite directions from the cell body, respectively. For instance, the bi-conical radiation is characteristic of bi-tufted and pyramidal cells of the cerebral cortex. Existence of such preferential directions of the dendritic radiation means breaking the spherical symmetry of the spatial distribution of the dendrites. A regular cone and paraboloid are geometrical figures of rotation, i.e. they are symmetrical relative to a certain straight line, the axis of rotation in the sense of equal extent from the axis in all directions determined by azimuthal angles. *Fan-type* radiation can be considered as an example of breaking the axial symmetry by putting restrictions on all azimuthal directions except those in a narrow

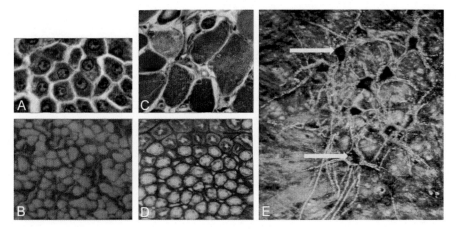

Fig 1.1

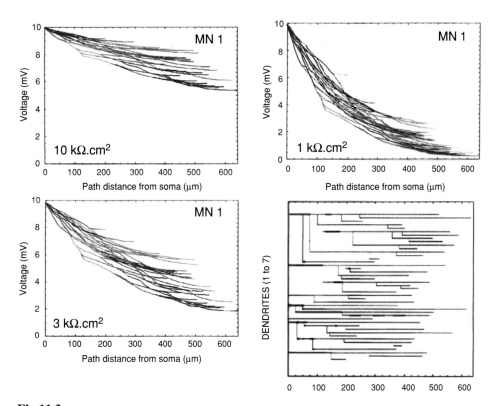

Fig 11.3

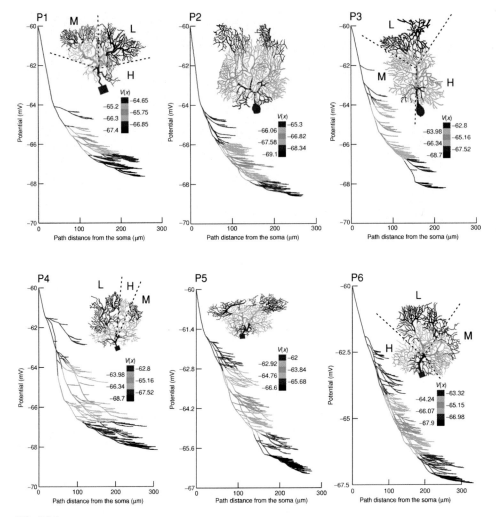

Fig 12.1

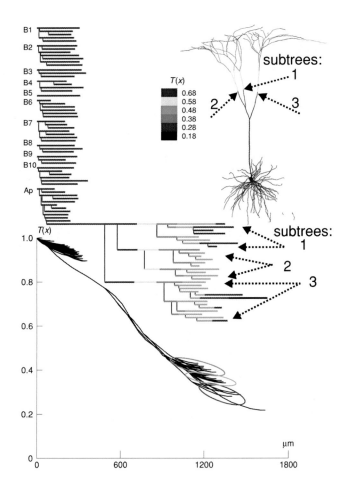

Fig 12.2

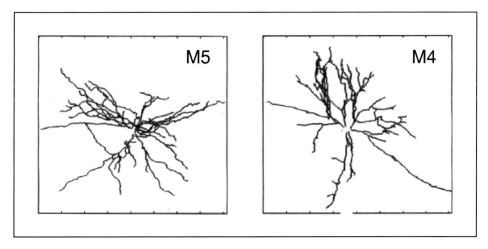

Fig 12.3

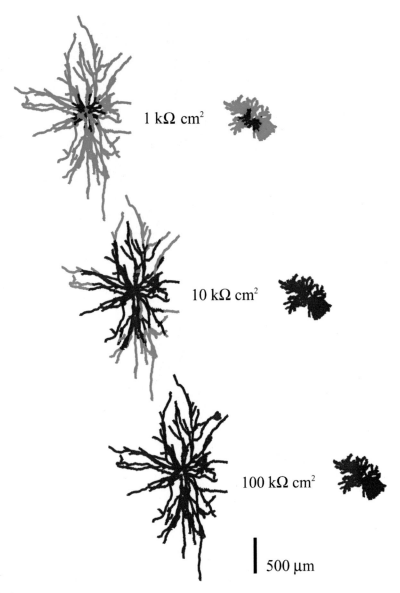

1 kΩ cm^2

10 kΩ cm^2

100 kΩ cm^2

500 μm

Fig 12.4

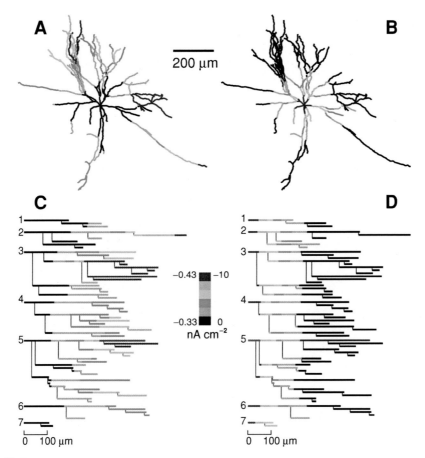

Fig 12.5

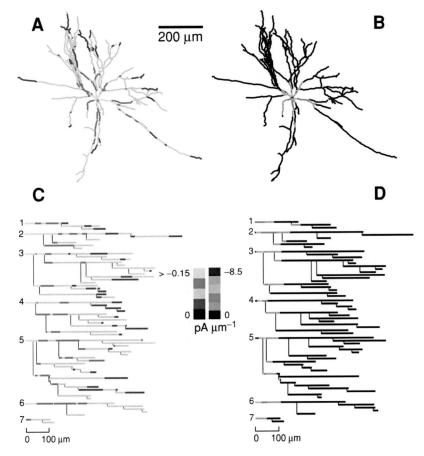

Fig 12.6

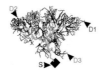

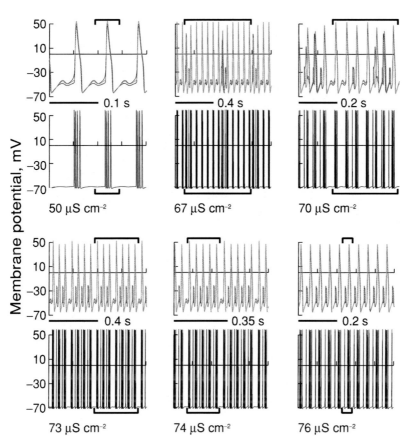

Fig 13.1

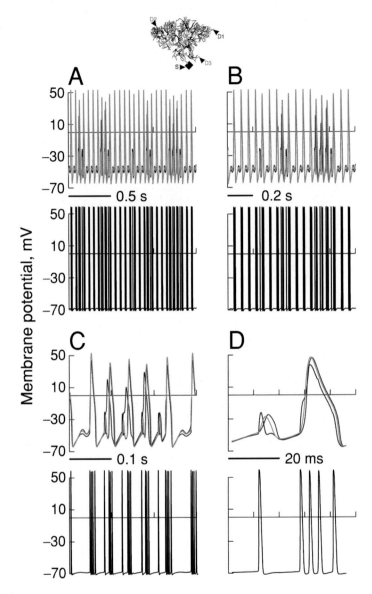

Fig 13.2

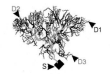

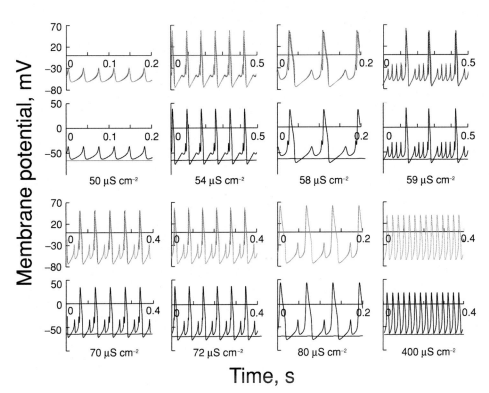

Membrane potential, mV

50 µS cm⁻²   54 µS cm⁻²   58 µS cm⁻²   59 µS cm⁻²

70 µS cm⁻²   72 µS cm⁻²   80 µS cm⁻²   400 µS cm⁻²

Time, s

Fig 13.3

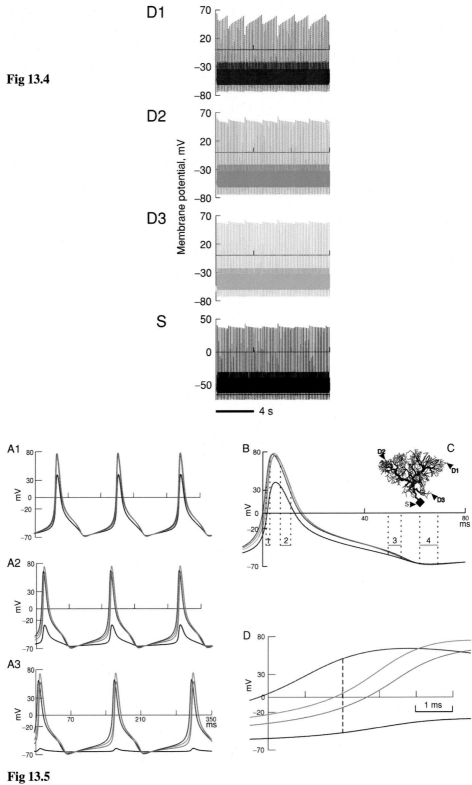

Fig 13.4

Fig 13.5

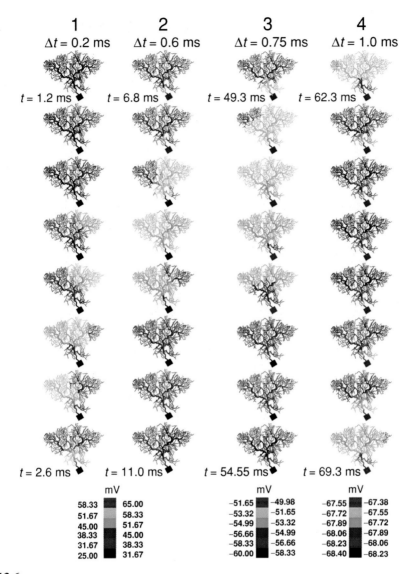

Fig 13.6

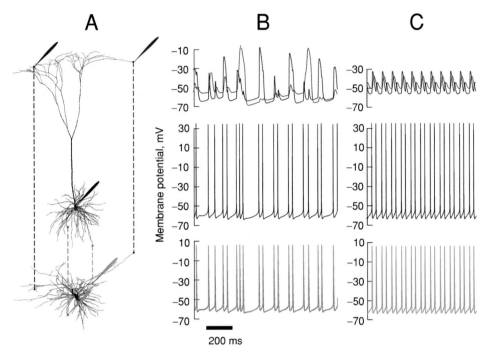

Fig 13.8

range that makes the dendritic field practically flat, like in the cerebellar Purkinje neurons.

The organization of dendrites in spatial angles centred at the soma provides information about how dendritic paths are trailed in the 3D peri-somatic space. The representation of the arborization in the 3D space shows the shape of the cell, its location and orientation relative to sources of its synaptic inputs and to other cells in the population. Although the 3D image of the arborization is widely used, there are many other important morphological details that are hardly visible. For instance, in the 3D image alone, it is hard to estimate and compare the lengths of the dendritic paths important for electrical computations, unlike their 3D orientation and extent. Longer paths may have longer extent in 3D (the so-called *air-way extent* measured by the length of the rectilinear segment between the soma and distal tip-dashed lines in Figure 9.1) if the spatial tortuosity of all curvilinear dendrites is not extensive, which is not always the case. In contrast, a tortuous long dendritic path may terminate at approximately the same or an even smaller air-way distance compared to a short and straight one.

A much clearer visualization of the spatial relationships between dendritic parts is provided by transformation of the corresponding 3D curves into rectified lines prolate in the same direction on the plane. Such a system of straight lines having the same length, thickness and connections as the dendritic branches is known as the dendrogram (Figure 9.1, left; see also Chapter 2). The dendrogram represents the dendritic space in two dimensions of a different nature. One dimension is continuous, measured by the coordinate x corresponding to the path distance from the soma. We travel along this dimension when moving along any dendritic path, as far as the dendritic paths extend. Another dimension is discrete: we travel along this dimension by making discrete jumps from one path to another, yet remaining at the same path distance from the soma. This dimension is measured by a set of discrete numbers corresponding to different paths. How far we move in this direction depends on the arborization complexity estimated by the complexity function, which counts the number of the dendritic paths at a given path distance x from the soma (Korogod *et al.*, 2000). Hence, the dendrogram provides a formal, discrete-continuous 2D space, on which one can map the electrical properties, e.g. parameters characterizing the distal-to-proximal (continuous) and path-to-path (discrete) relations. Noteworthy, a 2D dendrogram including diameters contains exhaustive morphological information required for computation of electrical processes in the dendrites. Due to one-to-one correspondence between the 2D dendrogram and 3D representations of the arborization one can re-map the computed properties from 2D to 3D representations and observe how they are organized in the 3D peri-somatic space.

9.2 Distinct 3D dendritic landscapes

Any classification of the dendritic structures in the 3D space is conditional and approximate. Due to richness of dendritic shapes one can meet many intermediate cases. However, representatives of clearly distinct classes could be a good choice for analysis of the 3D and 2D dendritic geometry and geometry-induced features of the electrical structures (Fiala and Harris, 1999). Attractive examples are arborizations, which occupy 3D regions of clearly different dimensions and symmetry:

- the flat, planar arborization of the Purkinje neurons of the cerebellum;
- the spherical arborization of motoneurons; and
- the bi-conical arborization of the pyramidal neurons of the cerebral cortex.

In the dendritic space of these neuron types, semi-schematically shown in Figure 9.2, one can distinguish characteristic 'landscape' parts, which can be attributed to the branching pattern classes introduced above for description of the whole arborization. This is the reason why the reconstructed Purkinje neurons, pyramidal neurons and motor neurons have been selected for our library of digitized cells used for the analysis of geometrical and electrical structures (see Section 9.3). What are the features of the 3D dendritic spaces of each selected type?

9.2.1 Planar dendritic field: Purkinje neurons

Purkinje neurons are characteristic and constant elements of the cerebellar cortex and have been described at length in numerous places (Llinás and Hillman, 1969). In the 3D space of the cerebellum, the Purkinje neurons are aligned like book pages or domino bricks stacked one in front of the other. The main morphological features of their dendritic space are depicted in Figure 9.2, A. The dendrites emerge from one or two short main stems and almost immediately give rise to secondary smooth branches which divide further to form a very dense plexus containing an enormous number of branchlets. The very complex arborization lies in one thin flat half-lunar layer (Figure 9.2, A). In the flat Purkinje neuron arborization, one can notice planar sectors (delimited by dashed lines), occupied by offspring radiating from the single main dendrite stem. The overlapping of the sectors belonging to different subtrees can be very small. Such a morphological structure of the dendritic space makes Purkinje neurons very convenient for mapping and studying spatial electrical phenomena. Hence, in future, description of the electrical structure of this type of dendritic field we will refer to planar sectors as structural components of the dendritic space.

A   B   C

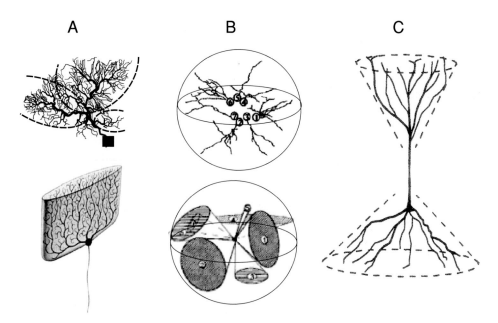

Figure 9.2 Schemata of the morphological dendritic spaces of a cerebellar Purkinje neuron (A), a brain stem abducens motoneuron (B) and a cortical pyramidal neuron (C). The flat dendritic field of the Purkinje neuron is partitioned into almost non-intersecting sectors (A, dashed lines) occupied by subtrees emerged from the main dendrite stem. The spherical dendritic field of abducens motoneuron (B) is partitioned between individual dendrites, which emerge from the soma and branch into practically non-intersecting cone-like regions. The dendritic field of the pyramidal neuron (C) is composed of the hemispheric basal part, the cylindrical part surrounding the main stem of apical dendrite with more or less numerous oblique subtrees and the disk-like part occupied by the apical dendrite tuft. Each of these parts is partitioned into spatial spherical or cylindrical sectors occupied by individual basal or oblique dendrites or by distal subtrees of the apical dendrite.

9.2.2 Spherical dendritic field: motor neurons

Sherrington (1952) called motoneurons *the final common path* because all the activity in the central nervous system that influences movement converges ultimately on motoneurons. The motoneurons are unique in that they are located in the central nervous system but project their axons outside to control muscles. They are among the most well-known and extensively studied neurons. All the dendrites of a single motoneuron scan a large peri-somatic space, each dendrite sweeping its own more or less extended sector. In the 3D space of the population, the branching regions of the neighbouring motoneurons overlap and this overlapping can be rather extensive.

Typically, the region of the peri-somatic 3D space occupied by the motoneuronal dendritic arborization is spherical (the 'spherical radiation pattern' according to classification of Fiala and Harris, 1999). Noteworthy is partition of the dendritic space of the motoneurons between individual dendrites. Arborizations of abducens motoneurons provide demonstrative examples (Bras *et al.*, 1987, 2003), one of which is illustrated in Figure 9.2, B. The space surrounding the soma of abducens motoneurons can be divided into conical (or paraboloid) spatial sectors owned by individual dendrites. Noteworthy, morphometrical analysis of this neuron type shows that a sector owned by a given dendrite does not intersect with the sectors owned by the neighbouring dendrites (Bras *et al.*, 1987, 2003). In our first work in 1987 (Bras *et al.*, 1987) one can find the results of detailed quantitative analysis of the dendritic geometry in 3D space of the population applied to one abducens and one laryngeal motoneuron of the cat. In these neurons, each dendrite characterized by 'computer dissection' is shown to occupy a definite field. A clear picture of their orientation is provided when each dendrite is represented separately. Their space occupancy is clearly different, as confirmed by the principal components analysis providing evidence that dendrites differ in their direction in space. Moreover, comparisons between dendrites made on the basis of length, diameter, tapering, branching pattern, daughter-branch ratio and branching power demonstrate that each single dendrite has its own personality. Further description of electrical structure of this type of dendritic field requires spatial sectors of certain 3D orientations.

9.2.3 Composite dendritic field: pyramidal neurons

The pyramidal neuron, called by Ramón y Cajal *the psychic cell*, is a multipolar neuron located in the hippocampus and cerebral cortex (Ramón y Cajal, 1911). These cells have a conically shaped soma, a single apical dendrite extending towards the pial surface, multiple basal dendrites and a single axon. In the primary motor cortex, layer V pyramidal cells are extremely large. The 3D space occupied by the pyramidal neuron dendrites is a composition of two or more parts and this partition is also conditional (Figure 9.2, C). According to the classification by Fiala and Harris (1999), the 3D dendritic radiation of the pyramidal neuron is classified as *bi-conical* with one conical region occupied by the apical arborization and another one by basal dendrites. However, the 'generatrix' is not a straight line for the apical or basal cone. For instance, the radii of the apical cone laid off from the apical stem as the axis in the distal tuft region are much greater than those in the proximal region, in which oblique dendrites radiate, and the axial length of the tuft region is much shorter than that of the pre-tuft stem. Because of this heterogeneity, one can consider the apical 3D space as composed of two parts: a nearly cylindrical region of oblique dendrites and early apical branching, and a disk-like or widely open cone-like region occupied by the tuft. If basal dendrites radiating at different angles relative to the vertical axis have very similar lengths, then the basal dendritic 3D space can be classified as hemispherical instead of conical. Whatever the division, each of the regions can be further divided into sectors, which give space to individual basal and oblique dendrites and to the apical subtrees (Figure 9.2, C). The apical dendrites spreading over two large regions of different 3D geometry and crossing several cortical layers are much longer than basal dendrites confined to a smaller peri-somatic region. This difference in the air-way extent is a pre-requisite for the metrical asymmetry of these two main dendrite types in terms of their path lengths. In the cortex 3D space, the pyramidal neurons are gathered in the cortical columns so called due to closely located parallel main stems of apical dendrites. It is not clear whether different positions of the pyramidal neurons in the column interior or periphery are associated with smaller or greater tangential branching asymmetry. This is the case for the crowns of botanical trees grown on the forest edge compared to those grown in the thicket. In the neocortical 'forest', such kinds of asymmetry are described in the layer IV stellate neurons (Lübke *et al.*, 2000). Further description of electrical structure of this type of dendritic field requires planar or volume (disk-like, cylindrical or spherical) sectors.

9.3 Digitized dendritic arborizations

The morphological structures of biological dendritic arborizations further used for computations of their electrical structures (Chapters 10–12) are collected in our library of digitized neurons, which are taken from different sources. They are neurons of the most well-known types that are characteristic of different parts of the central nervous system: cerebellar Purkinje neurons, neocortical pyramidal neurons and motoneurons of the brain stem and spinal cord. They have been recorded intracellularly, identified electro-physiologically, stained intracellularly with HRP and reconstructed as described in our corresponding work (Grant *et al.*, 1979; Durand *et al.*, 1983; Bras *et al.*, 1987; Durand, 1989; Bras *et al.*, 1993; Vigot and Batini, 1997, 1999; Korogod *et al.*, 2000; Kulagina *et al.*, 2007). The reconstructions of abducens motoneurons (Korogod *et al.*, 1994; Bras *et al.*, 2003), spinal motoneurons (Korogod *et al.*, 2000) and one of Purkinje neurons (Kulagina *et al.*, 2007) were performed at high spatial resolution. The spatial patterns of the dendritic arborizations of the library neurons (Figures 9.3–9.5) are representative of the classes to which they belong. Therefore, there are good reasons to extrapolate certain of their electrical properties to their class-mate neurons.

   In the context of this book, to consider the dendritic arborization as the deter-minant of its spatial electrical behaviour the most noteworthy structural fea-tures are the difference in size, the difference in complexity and especially the

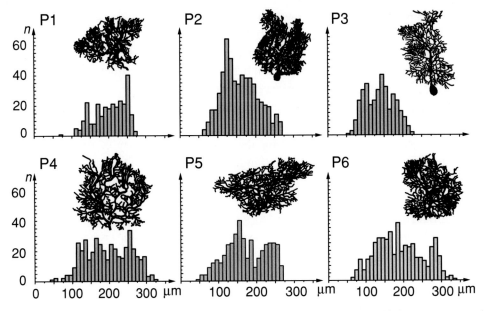

Figure 9.3 Reconstructed dendritic arborizations of cerebellar Purkinje neurons (P1 to P6) and their histograms of distribution of the dendritic path lengths as an indicator of metrical asymmetry. Abscissae: path distance from the soma, μm. Ordinates: number (*n*) or dendritic tips in a given interval of path lengths (bin width 10 μm). (Source: P1 from Kulagina *et al.*, 2007; P2 and P3 from Roth and Häusser, 2001; P4, P5 and P6 from Rapp *et al.*, 1994.)

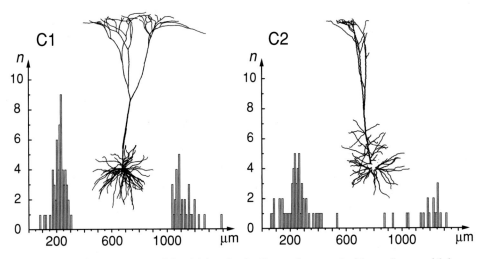

Figure 9.4 Reconstructed dendritic arborizations of neocortical layer 5 pyramidal neurons (C1 and C2) and their histograms of distribution of the dendritic path lengths as an indicator of metrical asymmetry. Abscissae: path distance from the soma, μm. Ordinates: number (n) or dendritic tips in a given interval of path lengths (bin width 10 μm). (Source: C1 from Mainen and Sejnowski, 1996; C2 from M. Larkum, University of Bern.)

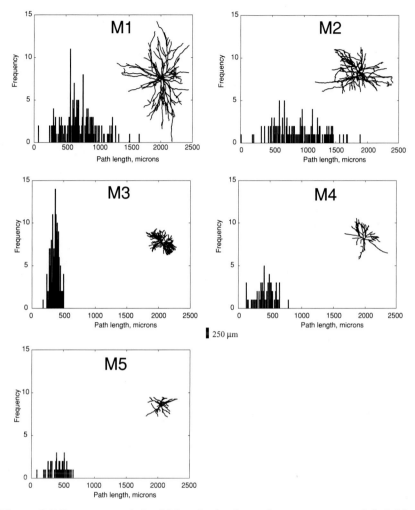

Figure 9.5 Reconstructed dendritic arborizations of motoneurons and their histograms of the distribution of the dendritic path lengths: spinal motoneurons of cat (M1), frog (M2) and rat (M3) and two abducens motoneurons of rat (M4 and M5). Abscissae: path distance from the soma, μm. Ordinates: number (*n*) or dendritic tips in a given interval of path lengths (bin width 10 μm). (From Korogod *et al.*, 1994, 2000.)

metrical asymmetry of the dendritic branching. The simplest, though not exhaustive, quantitative illustration of the metrical asymmetry of an arborization is provided by histograms of the distribution of the dendritic path lengths (Figures 9.3–9.5). In fact, the histogram shows the distribution of the path coordinates of distal tips of the dendrogram for each arborization.

9.3.1 Purkinje neurons

Six reconstructed cerebellar Purkinje neurons named P1 to P6 in our library (Figure 9.3) were selected from different sources. Neuron P1 reconstructed and fully analyzed in the work of Kulagina *et al.* (2007) was selected from a series of intracellularly labelled cells in slices of rat cerebellum (Vigot and Batini, 1997, 1999). The five other neurons, P2 to P6 were retrieved from publicly available databases as files importable into NEURON simulation software. Neurons P2 and P3 were described by Roth and Häusser (2001) as cells P19 and P20, respectively, and located at URL http://www.dendrite.org/dendritica?1.0/batchback/data/cells. Neurons P4, P5 and P6 were described by Rapp *et al.* (1994) as cell1, cell2 and cell3, respectively, and posted in the ModelDB database at URL http://senselab. med.yale.edu/senselab/modeldb/.

In this representative sample, the shortest dendritic paths have a length of about 50 µm and the longest ones are 250 to 350 µm long. The relatively short extent and small difference in length of individual dendritic paths account for a relatively small metrical asymmetry.

9.3.2 Neocortical pyramidal neurons

For our library we selected two reconstructed pyramidal neurons of layer 5 of rat neocortex (cells C1 and C1 in Figure 9.4). The neuron C1 published in Mainen and Sejnowski (1996) was retrieved from the open-access database ModelDB (file j4a.hoc at URL http://senselab.med.yale.edu/senselab/modeldb/ShowModel. asp?model=2488). The cell C2 was generously provided by Dr. Matthew Larkum, Department of Physiology, University of Bern.

The two neurons bear the features typical of their class: the long maximal extent of apical dendrites (up to 1300–1400 µm) and the large difference in path length (asymmetry) of apical and basal subtrees (Figure 9.4). The maximal path length of the basal dendrites reaches 300 µm, which is approximately as long as the extent of the whole Purkinje neuron arborization (cf. Figure 9.3). The minimal paths are about 50 µm.

9.3.3 Motoneurons

The five reconstructed motoneurons (M1 to M5 in Figure 9.5) are described in detail in our previous works (Korogod *et al.*, 1994, 2000). They were selected for the library on the basis of the morphological criteria as examples of cells with individual dendrites of different total lengths and widely varying morphometrical parameters. Three cells are spinal motoneurons of cat (M1), frog (M2) and young rat (M3) and two cells (M4 and M5) are abducens motoneurons of rat.

These motoneurons differ characteristically in the morphology of their dendritic spaces (Figure 9.5). The arborizations are composed of four dendrites in the frog motoneuron (M2), eight and seven in the rat abducens motoneurons (M4 and M5), ten in the rat spinal motoneuron (M3) and thirteen dendrites in the cat spinal motoneuron (M1). The total number of dendritic branches is the smallest in the rat abducens motoneuron (126) while this number is more than doubled in the spinal motoneuron of rat (282), frog (262) and cat (333). The total dendritic length is also the smallest in the rat abducens motoneuron (11,931 μm). Among the spinal motoneurons, the total dendritic length is the shortest in the rat (20,803 μm) while it is greater in the frog (52,411 μm) and the cat (59,557 μm). The total dendritic area follows the same rule, being the smallest in the rat abducens motoneuron (39,257 μm^2) and the largest in the spinal motoneurons with the largest surface area in the cat (301,738 μm^2). The index of complexity of each dendrite in the five motoneurons varies from 0 to 6.33. The highest complexity index (6.33) is found in one frog dendrite and the lowest (0) characterizes one dendrite in the frog and one in the rat abducens motoneuron. The coefficient of topological asymmetry varies in the range 0 to 0.75, being the highest in one dendrite of the rat abducens motoneuron. In this metrically very diversified sample, the same topology characterizes one trio and three pairs of dendrites in the five motoneurons (M1 to M5). Such dendrites have the same number of dendritic branches and the same branching patterns as indicated by equal topological asymmetry and/or complexity indexes (see Table 1 in Korogod *et al.*, 2000). Histograms of the path length distributions for the reconstructed motoneurons are shown in Figure 9.5.

References

Bras, H., Gogan, P. and Tyč-Dumont, S. (1987). The dendrites of single brain-stem motoneurons intracellularly labelled with horseradish peroxidase in the cat. Morphological and electrical differences. *Neuroscience*, **22**:947–970.

Bras, H., Korogod, S. M., Driencourt, Y., Gogan, P. and Tyč-Dumont, S. (1993). Stochastic geometry and electrotonic architecture of dendritic arborization of a brain-stem motoneuron. *Eur. J. Neurosci.*, **5**:1485–1493.

Bras, H., Lahjouji, F., Korogod, S. M., Kulagina, I. B. and Barbe, A. (2003). Heterogeneous synaptic covering and differential charge transfer sensitivity among the dendrites of a reconstructed abducens motor neurone: correlations between electron microscopic and computer simulation data. *J. Neurocytol.*, **32**:5–24.

Durand, J. (1989). Electrophysiological and morphological properties of rat abducens motoneurones. *Exp. Brain Res.*, **76**:141–152.

Durand, J., Gogan, P., Guéritaud, J., Horcholle-Bossavit, G. and Tyč-Dumont, S. (1983). Morphological and electrophysiological properties of trigeminal neurones projecting to the accessory abducens nucleus of the cat. *Exp. Brain Res.*, **53**:118–128.

Fiala, J. C. and Harris, K. M. (1999). Dendrite structure. In Stuart, G., Spruston, N. and Häusser, M. (eds.), *Dendrites*, p. 1–34, Oxford: Oxford University Press.

Grant, K., Guéritaud, J., Horcholle-Bossavit, G. and Tyč-Dumont, S. (1979). Morphological characteristics of lateral rectus motoneurones shown by intracellular injection of HRP. *J. Physiol. (Paris)*, **75**:513–519.

Korogod, S. M., Bras, H., Sarana, V. N., Gogan, P. and Tyč-Dumont, S. (1994). Electrotonic clusters in the dendritic arborization of abducens motoneurons of the rat. *Eur. J. Neurosci.*, **6**:1517–1527.

Korogod, S. M., Kulagina, I. B., Horcholle-Bossavit, G., Gogan, P. and Tyč-Dumont, S. (2000). Activity-dependent reconfiguration of the effective dendritic field of motoneurons. *J. Comp. Neurol.*, **422**:18–34.

Kulagina, I. B., Korogod, S. M., Horcholle-Bossavit, G., Batini, C. and Tyč-Dumont, S. (2007). The electro-dynamics of the dendritic space in Purkinje cells of the cerebellum. *Arch. Ital. Biol.*, **145**:211–233.

Llinás, R. and Hillman, D. E. (1969). Physiological and morphological organization of the cerebellar circuits in various vertebrates. In Llinás, R. (ed.), *Neurobiology of Cerebellar Evolution and Development*, p. 43–73, Chicago: AMA-ERF Institute for Biomedical Research.

Lübke, J., Egger, V., Sakmann, B. and Feldmeyer, D. (2000). Columnar organization of dendrites and axons of single and synaptically coupled excitatory spiny neurons in layer 4 of the rat barrel cortex. *J. Neurosci.*, **20**:5300–5311.

Mainen, Z. and Sejnowski, T. (1996). Influence of dendritic structure on firing pattern in model neocortical neurons. *Nature*, **382**:363–366.

Migliore, M. and Shepherd, G. M. (2005). Opinion: an integrated approach to classifying neuronal phenotypes. *Nat. Rev. Neurosci.*, **6**:810–818.

Ramón-Moliner, E. and Nauta, W. J. H. (1966). The iso-dendritic core of the brain stem. *J. Comp. Neurol.*, **126**:311–335.

Ramón y Cajal, S. (1911). *Histologie du Systéme Nerveux de l'Homme et des Vertébrés*, Paris: Maloine.

Rapp, M., Segev, Y. and Yarom, Y. (1994). Physiology, morphology and detailed passive models of guinea-pig cerebellar Purkinje cells. *J. Physiol.*, **474**:101–108.

Roth, A. and Häusser, M. (2001). Compartmental models of rat cerebellar Purkinje cells based on simultaneous somatic and dendritic patch-clamp recordings. *J. Physiol.*, **535**:445–472.

Sherrington, C. (1952). *The Integrative Action of the Nervous System*, London: Cambridge University Press.

Vigot, R. and Batini, C. (1997). GABA$_B$ receptor activation in Purkinje cells in cerebellar slices. *Neurosci. Res.*, **29**:151–160.

Vigot, R. and Batini, C. (1999). Purkinje cell inhibitory responses to 3-APPA (3-aminopropylphosphinic acid) in rat cerebellar slices. *Neurosci. Res.*, **34**:141–147.

10

Electrical structures of biological dendrites

Any live dendrite contains constitutive parts, such as the artificial elements used in Chapters 7 and 8 to demonstrate the biophysical laws that rule the proximal-to-distal and path-to-path electrical relationships. In fact, the live dendrite is made of similar elements and is ruled by the same laws. However, any piece of dendrite observed under a microscope in an histological preparation displays a much more complex shape than artificial elements. It appears tortuous, irregular, often nodular with branching points and daughter branches of different lengths and diameters. These idiosyncratic attributes are totally unpredictable, making dendrites unique.

In this chapter, as we tackle much more complex live objects, we consider first natural dendritic structures of moderate complexity: individual dendrites extracted from a whole arborization. We study electrical structures of natural dendrites in the same way as we did in the previous chapters dealing with simplified artificially built structures. We look for geometry-related features in the electrical structures in relation to structural heterogeneities and branchings in their natural occurrence. As the recognizable geometry-related features of electric structures are found for individual dendrites, they will be used as navigation tools in electrical structures of complex arborizations of different neuron types described in Chapter 11.

10.1 Geometry of an example dendrite

Here we show an example of a systematic study performed on one individual dendrite extracted from the reconstructed arborization of an abducens motoneuron of the rat (cell M5 in Figure 9.5). The location of the selected dendrite in the 3D space surrounding the soma is shown in Figure 10.1, A (Korogod *et al.*, 1998). The structural features important for shaping the electrical structure are hardly seen on this 3D image, which must be transformed into the dendrogram representation to display the branching pattern (the topology) and lengths of all branches and paths (Figure 10.1, B, top insert). From this representation, we get

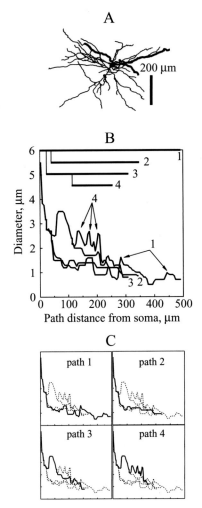

Figure 10.1 An individual dendrite taken from the reconstructed dendritic arborization of an abducens motoneuron of the rat (cell M5 in Figure 9.5): A: location of the selected dendrite (thick line) in the whole 3D arborization; B: the dendrogram (top insert) and heterogeneous diameter as a function of the path distance from soma along four dendritic paths (indicated by numbers 1 to 4) (Arrows point to featured variations of the diameter.); C: the diameter variation along each individual path. (Adapted from Korogod *et al.*, 1998.)

quantitative characteristics of the metrical asymmetry in terms of path lengths. Another important metrical parameter is the diameter. Its spatial variation is seen on a special plot of the whole dendrite (Figure 10.1, B) and in detail for all individual paths (Figure 10.1, C).

As one can clearly see in Figure 10.1, B and C, the selected dendrite has a moderately complex morphology with seven branches forming four paths. It is a sensible example in several respects. First, it is topologically symmetrical. The branch originating from the soma forms the first-order bifurcation and each sister branch emerging here forms the second-order bifurcation. Its topological asymmetry index is 0 (Verwer *et al.*, 1992). Second, this topologically symmetrical dendrite is metrically asymmetrical. Its metrical asymmetry is determined by the difference in lengths and diameters between paths. The longest path 1 is approximately 150 μm longer than its sister path 2 (this difference is about 1/3 of the longer sister branch's length). There is approximately the same 50 μm difference in length between the three progressively shorter paths 2, 3 and 4. In the second-order bifurcation of paths 2 and 4, the difference between the terminal branches is smaller in both absolute and relative values. The absolute difference is about 50 μm that makes about 1/4 of the longer branch length. Third, in the course of the reconstruction process, several increases in the dendritic diameter are observed along paths 1 and 4 (indicated by arrows in Figure 10.1). Although these swellings may well be artifacts due to intracellular injection of HRP, they are remarkable features that must be reflected in the electrical structure of the dendrite, according to our demonstration.

Let's attribute to this dendrite different membrane properties (passive or active) and synaptic inputs (single-site or distributed) to study its electrical structures and discover its geometry-induced electrical features.

10.2 Passive dendrite with single-site inputs

First, we compute the passive electrical structure represented by the path profiles of the relative effectiveness of the somatopetal current transfer $T(x)$. Figure 10.2 shows such an electrical structure computed for the specific membrane resistance $R_m = 3\,k\Omega \cdot cm^2$ and the cytoplasm resistivity $R_i = 100\,\Omega \cdot cm$.

As expected, the somatopetal current transfer effectiveness $T(x)$ decays with the path distance from the soma, with unequal rates along the asymmetrical paths. The decay is smooth along uniform segments, but not at the sites of abrupt change in the diameter or branching. At bifurcations, the slopes of decay along asymmetrical sister branches are different and the corresponding branching path profiles of $T(x)$ diverge. Resulting from such a divergence, the values of $T(x)$ are unequal at sites which are equidistant from the soma, but located on different dendritic paths. The divergence of the path profiles is greater if the difference between the paths in their length (*the metrical asymmetry*) is great. In our example, the difference in length is small between the sister paths 2 and 3 and is much greater when either of these paths are compared to the longest path 1. Correspondingly, the $T(x)$ profile along path 1 deviates greatly from those along paths 2 and 3. On the path 1 profile of $T(x)$ one can clearly see variations of the slope at the path distances corresponding to

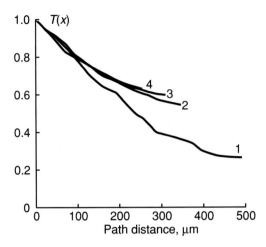

Figure 10.2 Passive electrical structure of the individual dendrite of rat abducens motoneuron shown in Figure 10.1. Abscissa: path distance from the soma, μm. Ordinate: the relative current transfer effectiveness, dimensionless.

large variations of the dendritic diameter (cf. Figure 10.1, B, C). These geometry-induced features of the passive electrical structure expressed in terms of $T(x)$ can now be used as a reference to consider other types of electrical structures.

10.3 Dendrites with distributed inputs

10.3.1 Dendrite with positive I–V relation slope

Now we apply homogeneously distributed tonic synaptic activation to this dendrite. We keep the same homogeneous membrane properties (passive or Hodgkin–Huxley-type active) with the same set of electrical parameters as in the case of the simplest artificial structures (Chapters 7 and 8). Correspondingly, the steady-state local I–V relations of the dendritic membrane remain the same: linear or non-linear, each with positive slope over the whole range of membrane voltages.

Introducing a steady, spatially homogeneous, excitatory conductivity to the dendrite with either passive or active membranes produces inhomogeneous steady voltages and currents (Figure 10.3, A and E, solid lines). The transmembrane depolarization $E(x)$ is the greatest at the distal tips and decays toward the soma and further to the distal axon end. Noteworthy, the path profiles of $E(x)$ look like mirror images of the path profiles of $T(x)$ considered in the previous section (Figure 10.2). The effective equilibrium potential $E_q(x)$ remains at the initial level −65 mV in the soma and axon, but is shifted to depolarization in the dendritic branches. It is homogeneous ($E_q = -32.5$ mV) throughout all paths of the passive dendrite (dashed line in Figure 10.3, A) with homogeneous $G_s = G_{p,d}$ and $G_m = G_s + G_{p,d}$

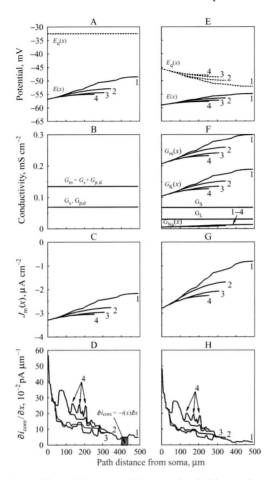

Figure 10.3 Path profiles of the potentials, conductivities and currents resulting from steady uniform activation of excitatory synaptic inputs distributed along the individual dendrite with passive (A–D) or active (E–H) extra-synaptic membranes. Abscissae: path distance from soma, μm. Ordinates (A, E): transmembrane potential $E(x)$ (solid lines) and effective equilibrium potential of the total transmembrane current $E_q(x)$ (dashed lines), mV; (B): homogeneous total membrane conductivity G_m and its equal partial conductivities of synaptic and passive extra-synaptic dendritic membrane (G_s and $G_{p,d}$), mS cm^{-2}; (F): inhomogeneous total membrane conductivity $G_m(x)$ with its inhomogeneous voltage-dependent ($G_{Na}(x)$ and $G_K(x)$) and homogeneous voltage-independent (G_s and G_L) components, mS cm^{-2}; (C, G): total membrane current density per unit membrane area $J_m(x)$, μA cm^{-2}; (D, H): core current increment $\partial i_{core}/\partial x = -i(x)$ equal to minus the total current per unit path length, pA μm^{-1}. Striped area in D: current collected from the path element ∂x. Numbers 1–4 indicate the paths shown on the dendrogram in Figure 10.1, B. (From Korogod *et al.*, 1998.)

(Figure 10.3, B). However, $E_q(x)$ is inhomogeneous in the active dendrite; it is maximal at the proximal end and decays with different rates towards the distal tips (Figure 10.3, E, dashed lines). The active membrane conductivity $G_m(x)$ increases with increasing path distances from the soma (Figure 10.3, F). Its voltage-independent components G_s and G_L are homogeneous, whereas voltage-dependent ones $G_{Na}(x)$ and $G_K(x)$ follow inhomogeneous membrane depolarization $E(x)$. The main contribution comes from the non-inactivating potassium conductivity $G_K(x)$ associated with hyperpolarization equilibrium potential E_K. The inactivating sodium conductivity $G_{Na}(x)$ associated with depolarization equilibrium potential E_{Na} gives a one order of magnitude smaller contribution. With such profiles of $E(x)$ and $E_q(x)$, the driving potential $E(x) - E_q(x)$ is negative and decreases with path distance from the soma, with a greater rate in the active case. In both passive and active dendrites, the surface density of the dendritic current monotonically decreases with increasing path distance from the soma (Figure 10.3, C and G). The increment of the somatopetal core current, which is minus the membrane current density per unit length $\partial i_{core}(x)/\partial x = -i(x) = -\pi \cdot D(x) \cdot J_m(x)$ also decreases but not monotonically (Figure 10.3, D and H).

Abrupt elevations of the plot are observed on some dendritic segments. Comparison with the path profiles of the dendritic diameters $D(x)$ (Figure 10.1, B, C) shows that they correspond to the segments with abrupt increased diameters. Thus, the sites that are more distal give progressively smaller contributions to the core current. However, if a local increase in the diameter occurs and is greater than the decrease in the surface current density, the contribution to the core current increases at this location. The path profiles of spatially inhomogeneous characteristics along asymmetrical sister branches and paths diverge. As in Section 8.3.1 (see also Korogod and Kulagina, 1998), comparison of equidistant sites $x = x_{long} = x_{short}$ on paths of different length (e.g. long path 1 and short path 2) shows, on the shorter path: (i) smaller $E(x)$; (ii) greater active $E_q(x)$; (iii) greater driving potential $E(x) - E_q(x)$; (iv) greater current density $J_m(x)$ and (v) greater relative effectiveness of passive somatopetal current transfer from single-site sources $T(x)$ (Bras *et al.*, 1993). Finally, (vi) an elementary contribution to the somatopetal core current from distributed sources is greater if the ratio of the diameters $D(x_{long})/D(x_{short})$ do not exceed the ratio of the current densities $J_m(x_{short})/J_m(x_{long})$.

From these findings, it becomes obvious that the type of distal-to-proximal relation is determined by the type of local *I–V* relation in the dendrite in both passive and active configurations. Thus, whatever the configuration of the dendritic membrane, the natural geometry specifies this general spatial relation according to lengths and heterogeneous diameters along different paths. The metrical asymmetry of the dendritic paths receiving distributed tonic activation brings about a clear segregation of the path profiles of the transmembrane voltage and, if present, of the voltage-dependent conductances, of the effective equilibrium potential $E_q(x)$ and of the surface density $J_m(x)$ of the total membrane current. The path profiles along the most asymmetrical path 1 are the most different from other profiles. Conversely, the path profiles are close to each other in the second-order bifurcation of small metrical asymmetry composed of paths 3 and 4. The varying dendritic diameter is another contributor to metrical asymmetry. It remarkably modulates the core current increment per unit path length and therefore the contribution of the corresponding dendritic sites to the total current delivered along the path to the soma.

10.3.2 Dendrite with an N-shaped I–V relation

The same dendrite is used with the other type of *I–V* relation of the dendritic membrane (Korogod *et al.*, 2002). We take the same cocktail of dendritic conductances including passive extra-synaptic and active NMDA-type synaptic components which produces electrical bistability in artificial dendrites as described in Section 8.3.2. The protocol of simulations is also the same. However, for inducing electrical bistability in the reconstructed dendrite, we have to set an intensity of synaptic activation different from that used in the case of the artificial dendrite.

The biophysical mechanisms defining the somatopetal current transfer effectiveness are examined in the two stable steady states of low and high depolarization (the *downstate* and *upstate*), inherent in the bistability. The computations are performed at two maximum synaptic conductivities $\overline{G}_{NMDA} = 8.9$ mS cm^{-2} (Figure 10.4, A1–D1) and $\overline{G}_{NMDA} = 9.0$ mS cm^{-2} (Figure 10.4, A2–D2), which are just below and above the upper limit of the electrical bistability for this dendrite. Four electrical parameters are plotted: the transmembrane potential and the effective equilibrium potential of the total membrane current (Figure 10.4, A1 and A2); the total membrane conductivity and its synaptic component (Figure 10.4, B1 and B2); the membrane current per unit area (Figure 10.4, C1 and C2) and the core current increment per unit path length (Figure 10.4, D1 and D2), expressed as a function of the path distance from the soma. Each parameter can thus be related to the four dendritic branches, their length, their asymmetry and variations in their diameters.

In the *downstate*, all four parameters are extremely sensitive to the local geometry of the dendritic branches (Figure 10.4, A1–D1). The four dendritic paths (1 to 4) are clearly differentiated by their transmembrane potential $E(x)$ with divergent profiles at branching points. The greater the asymmetry of the branching, the greater the divergence of the voltage profiles. The dendritic depolarization reaches unequal maximum levels at the four distal tips (Figure 10.4, A1) and decays with unequal rates along the asymmetrical paths. The total membrane conductivity $G_m(x)$ is also

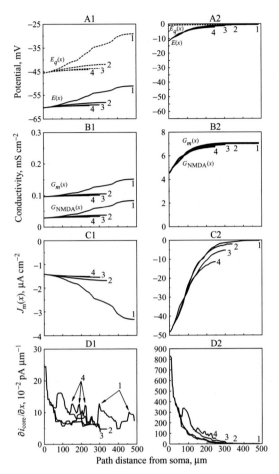

Figure 10.4 Impact of dendritic geometry on path profiles of electrical parameters in a dendrite with an N-shaped I–V relation. The electrical bistability is induced by tonic activation of distributed NMDA-type glutamatergic synaptic conductance. Computations are performed at two synaptic intensities, $\overline{G}_{NMDA} = 8.9\ \text{mS cm}^{-2}$ (row A1–D1) and $\overline{G}_{NMDA} = 9.0\ \text{mS cm}^{-2}$ (row A2–D2), corresponding to values below and above the upper limit of the range of electrical bistability for this dendrite. The electrical parameters are shown along paths 1 to 4 of the dendrite as a function of the path distance from the soma. Abscissae: path distance from soma, μm. Ordinates (A1, A2): The transmembrane potential $E(x)$ and the effective equilibrium potential of the total transmembrane current $E_q(x)$. (B1, B2): The total membrane conductance per unit membrane area $G_m(x)$ and its active synaptic component $G_{NMDA}(x)$. (C1, C2): The total current per unit membrane area $J_m(x)$. (D1, D2): The core current increment per unit path length $\partial i_{core}(x)/\partial x$. (From Korogod *et al.*, 2002.)

spatially heterogeneous (Figure 10.4, B1) and follows the profile of the membrane potential (Figure 10.4, A1). The synaptic conductivity $G_{NMDA}(x)$ is of the same order of magnitude as the passive extra-synaptic conductivity and makes up about $1/3$ to $1/2$ of the total membrane conductivity $G_m(x)$ at the root and the distal tip of path 1. The total current density per unit membrane area $J_m(x)$ (Figure 10.4, C1) is the product of the total membrane conductivity $G_m(x)$ (Figure 10.4, B1) and the driving potential $E(x) - E_q(x)$ in Figure 10.4, A1. The absolute value of $J_m(x)$ increases from 1.4 to 3.4 μA cm^{-2} with the path distance from the soma. The largest increase concerns the longest and most depolarized path 1. The core current increment per unit path length $\partial i_{core}/\partial x$ is calculated as the product of $J_m(x)$ taken with the opposite sign and the dendritic perimeter $\pi D(x)$. The core current decreases sharply over the first 50 μm in the four dendritic paths and then fluctuates over a narrow range (0.07 to 0.12 pA μm^{-1}) according to the variations of the dendritic diameters (Figure 10.1, B, C), reflecting accurately these structural heterogeneities.

In the *upstate*, the four electrical parameters behave in a totally different way. The transmembrane potentials are similar in the four dendritic paths, with steep slopes in their proximal parts, and reach saturation near the reversal potential of the synaptic current after the first 200 μm from the soma (Figure 10.4, A2). Similarly, the synaptic conductivity $G_{NMDA}(x)$ is nearly identical in the four dendritic paths (Figure 10.4, B2) and more than one order of magnitude greater than in the low depolarization state (downstate). It should be noted that, with NMDA conductances close to the upper limit for electrical bistability, the membrane depolarization exceeds the values recorded experimentally from the soma of live neurons. Decreasing synaptic conductivity below this limit or clamping the soma at a lower membrane potential brings the membrane depolarization close to experimental values and does not alter the fundamental behaviour of the model. Using this upper limit is justified by the fact that it provides extreme conditions in which the most contrasted patterns can be illustrated. The inward current density (Figure 10.4, C2) decreases with the path distance from the soma in all four dendritic paths with a sharp slope in their most proximal parts to reach zero in their distal parts (> 400 μm from the soma). There, the synaptic conductivity is very high and the driving potential is zero as the membrane depolarization $E(x)$ saturates close to the reversal potential of the synaptic current $E_{NMDA} = 0$ mV. It is remarkable that the total current density orders the four dendritic paths in the sequence No. 4 < No. 3 < No. 2 < No. 1 in the downstate but in the opposite sequence No. 1 < No. 2 < No. 3 < No. 4 in the upstate. The core current in each dendritic path (Figure 10.4, D2) decreases sharply over the first 300 μm from the soma to reach zero in their distal parts, indicating that the periphery of the dendrite does not contribute to the total somatopetal current.

The modulatory effect of the dendritic diameter heterogeneity on the core current increment (longitudinal transfer effectiveness from distributed sources) is also more prominent in the downstate. In the upstate, only the large proximal heterogeneity preceding second-order bifurcation of paths 3 and 4 has this impact, whereas the distal parts of the dendrite are all equally ineffective. The metrical asymmetry of branching also causes the divergence of electrical path profiles, which is most prominent in the downstate and very small in the upstate. The greater asymmetry of paths, the more segregated the path profiles are. This is clearly demonstrated by the greatest divergence of electrical profiles along the most asymmetrical path 1. The profiles along the other paths form a more compact group.

We conclude that the N-shaped type of $I–V$ relation of the reconstructed dendrite determines the type of the distal-to-proximal relation along the dendritic paths. If the membrane depolarization is within the range of positive slope of the $I–V$ relation, then a smaller inward current is generated at greater depolarization as in the previous case (Section 8.3.2). However, if the depolarization is within the range of the negative slope, then a greater depolarization generates a greater inward current density. In both upstate and downstate, the dendritic depolarization is higher in the more distal regions. In the downstate, the depolarization over the whole dendrite is within the range of the negative $I–V$ slope and, correspondingly, the inward current density is greater in the more depolarized distal regions. The spatial relation is opposite in the upstate since the depolarization is now within the range of the positive slope. In this state, more depolarized distal regions generate inward currents of smaller density.

Our detailed analysis of the electrical profile of the single live dendrites demonstrates that its specific geometry rules the path-to-path electrical relations whatever the membrane properties, passive or active.

10.4 Reconfigurations of passive electrical structures

In the previous sections, attention has focused on the electrical consequences of the metrical asymmetry and some other important aspects have been cast aside. We must also consider the impact of the size of the dendrites. Indeed, the dendrites of different neurons differ in their path distance extents. Another important aspect is the dependence of the geometry-related electrical structure on the electrical parameters, first of all on the membrane resistivity, which may change, e.g. as a result of changing the intensity of synaptic activation. Here we consider these aspects with the example of a pair of metrically different individual dendrites with equal topology extracted from arborizations of significantly different sizes. These are the dendrite 5 of the rat (M3) and the dendrite 6 of the cat (M1) spinal motoneurons (Figure 9.5 and see Chapter 9). Both dendrites have the same number

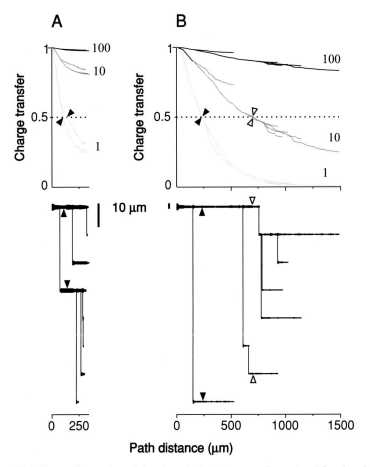

Figure 10.5 Reconfiguration of the electrical structures of two dendrites by changing R_m. Top: Somatopetal charge transfer effectiveness $T(x)$ (ordinates) computed as a function of the path distance from soma (abscissae) under $R_m = 100 \, k\Omega \cdot cm^2$ (black lines), $10 \, k\Omega \cdot cm^2$ (dark grey) and $1 \, k\Omega \cdot cm^2$ (light grey). Arrowheads indicate dendritic sites with $T(x) = 0.5$ defining the outer borders of the high efficiency domains. Bottom: Dendrograms of dendrite 5 (A) and dendrite 6 (B) with the same number of branches (seven) and the same asymmetry index (0.57) but different metrical characteristics. The same arrowheads on dendrites delimitate the distal borders of the high efficiency domains on the dendritic paths. (From Korogod *et al.*, 2000.)

of branches (seven) and the same topological asymmetry index (0.57), but they display very different metrical parameters. The path lengths vary from 250 to 345 μm in the rat and from 500 to 1477 μm in the cat. The cumulative path length of the branches is 3.5 times smaller in the rat than in the cat dendrite. The diameters of the stem dendrites and their evolutions along the dendritic paths are also different (Figure 10.5, lower part).

The passive electrical structure of each dendrite is represented by $T(x)$ profiles computed for three uniform specific membrane resistances $R_m = 100$, 10 and $1\,k\Omega \cdot cm^2$ (Figure 10.5, upper part).

Both dendrites under each R_m show the general features of the somatopetal charge transfer effectiveness $T(x)$ decay with path distance from the soma as described above. The decaying path profiles of $T(x)$ along asymmetrical paths diverge. At any given dendritic site x, $T(x)$ decreases as the values of R_m decrease from 100 to 10 and $1\,k\Omega \cdot cm^2$. Correspondingly, the path distances to the dendritic sites of a given effectiveness $T(x)$ decrease with R_m. Spatially homogeneous, equal decrements in the membrane resistivity produce spatially inhomogeneous and unequal decrements in $T(x)$. These coupled geometry- and R_m-dependent changes in the charge transfer effectiveness domain are qualitatively similar for any level of $T(x)$.

Consider now two aspects of the same picture. First, we fix a certain $T(x)$ level and look for locations x on different dendritic paths that have the same effectiveness. This is illustrated in Figure 10.5 in which the reference level is arbitrarily fixed at $T(x) = 0.5$ (horizontal dashed line). The dendritic branches of the two dendrites are divided into two domains of different efficiency, one higher and one lower than $T(x) = 0.5$. The arrowheads in Figure 10.5 indicate the dendritic sites with $T(x) = 0.5$ defining the outer border of the high-efficiency domains. These border sites are not equidistant on different dendritic paths. The shorter rat dendrite is highly efficient over its whole extent at $R_m = 100$ and $10\,k\Omega \cdot cm^2$, but not at $1\,k\Omega \cdot cm^2$, where distal 125 μm and longer segments are in the low efficiency domain (Figure 10.5 A, arrows). The longer cat dendrite is highly efficient over its whole extent at $100\,k\Omega \cdot cm^2$ but not at 10 and $1\,k\Omega \cdot cm^2$ (Figure 10.5, B) where large distal segments reduce their effectiveness to below the 0.5 level. Second, we fix a certain path distance x and consider the difference in the values of $T(x)$ at equidistant locations x on different dendritic paths. A noteworthy observation is that $T(x)$ divergence is observed for different values of the passive membrane resistivity R_m (or the inverse value, the conductivity $G_m = 1/R_m$). The divergence is the greatest in the medium range of $R_m = 1/G_m$ and smaller in the high- and low-resistance ranges (low- and high-conductance ranges). The medium R_m range providing the greatest $T(x)$ divergence is size-specific: the longer the dendrites, the greater the R_m values inducing the maximum divergence. In our example, the $T(x)$ profiles along the asymmetrical branches of the longer dendrite of the cat motoneuron diverge significantly at about one order of magnitude greater R_m compared to the shorter rat motoneuron dendrites. In the cat dendrite, the significant fact is that the shortest branch is more efficient at 100 and $10\,k\Omega \cdot cm^2$ than its much longer sister branch, but becomes less effective at $1\,k\Omega \cdot cm^2$.

References

Bras, H., Korogod, S., Driencourt, Y., Gogan, P. and Tyč-Dumont, S. (1993). Stochastic geometry and electrotonic architecture of dendritic arborization of a brain-stem motoneuron. *Eur. J. Neurosci.*, **5**:1405–1493.

Korogod, S. M. and Kulagina, I. B. (1998). Geometry-induced features of current transfer in neuronal dendrites with tonically activated conductances. *Biol. Cybern.*, **79**:231–240.

Korogod, S. M., Kulagina, I., Horcholle-Bossavit, G., Gogan, P. and Tyč-Dumont, S. (2000). Activity-dependent reconfiguration of the effective dendritic field of motoneurons. *J. Comp. Neurol.*, **442**:18–34.

Korogod, S. M., Kulagina, I. B., Kukushka, V. I., Gogan, P. and Tyč-Dumont, S. (2002). Spatial reconfiguration of charge transfer effectiveness in active bistable dendritic arborizations. *Eur. J. Neurosci.*, **16**:2260–2270.

Korogod, S. M., Kulagina, I. B. and Tyč-Dumont, S. (1998). Transfer properties of neuronal dendrites with tonically activated conductances. *Neurophysiology*, **30**:203–207.

Verwer, R. W. H., Van Pelt, J. and Uylings, H. B. M. (1992). An introduction to topological analysis of neurones. In Stewart, M. G. (ed.), *Quantitative Methods in Neuroanatomy*, p. 295–323, New-York: John Wiley & Sons, Inc.

11

Electrical structure of the whole arborization

The superposition of the electrical profiles of all individual dendrites of a given neuron represents the electrical structure of the whole arborization. The electrical path profiles form a complex tree-like structure that is topologically equivalent (homeomorphous) to the morphological dendritic arborization as both of them are composed of the same number of identically connected branches and paths. Due to this one-to-one correspondence between the dendritic paths and their electrical profiles, the tree-like electrical structure acquires several important features of the morphological tree such as branching pattern, path distance extent and complexity function.

Which new aspects are brought in when several individual dendrites are united in the whole arborization? Although one can expect occurrence or absence of new properties induced by the whole system, we focus on the new emerging properties in this chapter.

To find out what is the case, we explore the whole arborization electrical structure by applying the same protocols in the same sequence (passive membrane and single-site inputs, passive or active membrane and distributed inputs) as those applied to individual dendrites in the preceding section. Namely, we start with the passive electrical structure of the whole arborization represented by the superposition of the current transfer profiles $T(x)$ of individual dendrites, which remain the same as those computed for each extracted individual dendrite.

11.1 Organization of the spatial electrical profiles

We start by computing passive electrical structures of the whole arborization transferring single-site inputs for different neurons. The careful observation of the patterns of spatial electrical profiles reveals two main organizations. Depending on the dominating pattern of the mutual locations of the diverging profiles, we classify these organizations as *continuum-type* or *cluster-type*.

The electrical structure of the small dendritic arborization of a spinal motoneuron of a young rat (cell M3 in Figure 9.5) provides an example of the continuum-type (Figure 11.1) The diverging electrical profiles of individual dendrites intermingle and densely cover the plane of the plot, resembling a comet tail. The density is high in the middle of the 'tail' with occasional profiles above and below the main stream.

This arrangement corresponds to the histogram of the distribution of the dendritic path lengths having a clear narrow single mode with a small number of distinctly shorter and longer paths (Figure 9.5). Hence, small metrical asymmetry favours the continuum-type organization of electrical profiles.

A remarkably different type of passive electrical structure is provided by the dendritic arborizations of Purkinje and pyramidal neurons (library cells P1 and C1, Chapter 9) shown in Figure 11.2. In each studied case, the electrical profiles are organized in bundles separated by 'empty' space in which no or few profiles are found. The bundles are defined as sets of dendritic branches that display similar electrical transfer properties at given distances from the soma. As we know from the analysis of electrical structure of artificial bifurcations (Chapters 7 and 8), the proximity of electrical profiles indicate similarity of electrical transfer properties $T(x)$ of the corresponding sister paths with small metrical asymmetry. The arborization is characterized by a number of bundles, indicating similarity of electrical properties of the branches. Conversely, distinct bundles indicate between-group dissimilarity of electrical properties of the corresponding dendritic paths. Hence, the passive electrical structure of the whole reconstructed arborization is informative with regard to the presence of dendritic domains similar or dissimilar in their transfer properties. Comparing the bundles of electrical profiles and the corresponding dendrograms (Figure 11.2), two important facts must be underlined. Some bundles (indicated by open arrows) reflect the asymmetry between the subtrees belonging to the same individual dendrite: to the unique dendrite of the Purkinje neuron (left) or to the apical dendrite of the neocortical pyramidal neuron (right). The asymmetry between different individual dendrites has the most distinct impact on the electrical structure of the whole arborization of the neocortical pyramidal neuron: the dense bundle corresponding to the basal dendrites (black arrow) is clearly distinct from the bundles corresponding to the apical tuft (open arrows). This is in good correspondence with the remarkable difference between these groups of dendrites in their path lengths, as is clearly seen on the dendrogram below and quantitatively characterized by the histogram in Figure 9.4, in which the mode of shorter basal dendrites is far apart from that of the much longer apical paths. We classify this

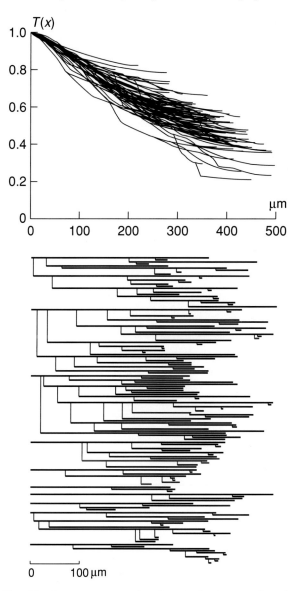

Figure 11.1 Top: Continuum-type passive electrical structure of a spinal motoneuron of young rat. The electrical structure is represented by the current transfer effectiveness $T(x)$ as a dimensionless function of the path distance x from the soma (abscissa, μm) computed at $G_m = 350\,\mu\text{S}\,\text{cm}^{-2}$ and $R_i = 100\,\Omega\cdot\text{cm}$. Bottom: The dendrogram of the whole reconstructed arborization illustrating the metrical asymmetry due to differences in length between the dendritic paths (see also the histogram in Figure 9.5). The dendritic diameters are not shown.

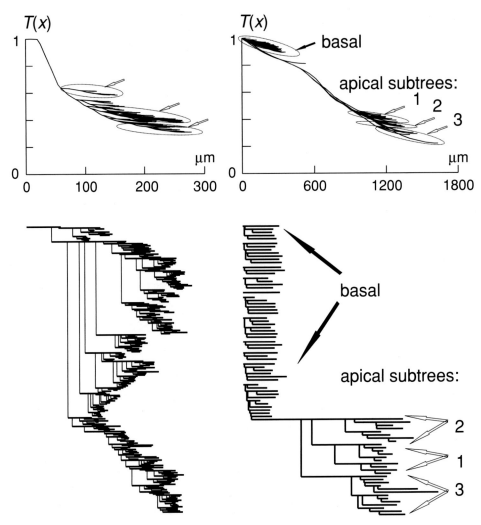

Figure 11.2 Top: Cluster-type passive electrical structures of Purkinje neuron P1 (left) and neocortical pyramidal neuron C1 (right). The electrical structure is represented by the current transfer effectiveness $T(x)$ as a dimensionless function of the path distance x from the soma (abscissa, μm) computed at $G_m = 300 \, \mu S \, cm^{-2}$ and $R_i = 250 \, \Omega \cdot cm$ for P1, and at $G_m = 40 \, \mu S \, cm^{-2}$ and $R_i = 150 \, \Omega \cdot cm$ for C1. The arrows indicate bundles of electrical profiles with similar $T(x)$. Bottom: The dendrogram of the whole reconstructed arborization of the corresponding neurons illustrating the metrical asymmetry due to differences in length between the dendritic paths (see also the histograms in Figures 9.3 and 9.4). The dendritic diameters are not shown.

organization as cluster-type, signifying the presence of multiple dendritic elements with similar patterns of metrical asymmetry.

11.1.1 An electrical detector of metrical asymmetry

In Chapters 7 and 8, we noticed that the passive electrical transfer function $T(x)$ is a good sensor of individual structural heterogeneities in the dendritic structure, such as abrupt variations in the diameter or asymmetrical branching. Now we use the same tool as an electrical detector of the collective asymmetrical properties characteristic of groups of dendritic elements. In this context, gathering the electrical profiles into groups deserves special attention, especially a new emerging property not predicted, where the metrical asymmetry between the dendritic paths is not clearly distinct. This property opens new possibilities for detecting metrical asymmetry patterns based on the analysis of the electrical profiles.

Let's consider first the passive electrical structure of the Purkinje neuron computed with $G_m = 300\,\mu S\,cm^{-2}$ (Figure 11.2, left). First, the distinction of the groups of electrical profiles points out the presence of significant metrical asymmetry of the dendritic paths in the arborization. If the asymmetry causes electrical distinction, then the electrical distinction detects the existence of significant asymmetry. Second, the fact that the profiles form distinct bundles means that metrical asymmetry pattern is repetitive: each repeating instance of significant asymmetry contributes repetitively to the distinct groups, making them more numerous. In this case, natural variability of path length and diameters (variability of the metrical asymmetry) is unable to dissipate the bundles of profiles into a continuum. In short, to have distinct groups of electrical profiles, the arborization must have significantly asymmetrical branchings and similar branchings must be numerous. These are pre-requisites for the bundled electrical structure of the Purkinje neuron arborization at high conductivity (low resistivity) of the passive dendritic membrane ($G_m = 300\,\mu S\,cm^{-2}$).

The geometry of the dendritic arborization of the pyramidal neuron is noticeable in two respects: the asymmetry between basal and apical dendrites and that between subtrees within the apical dendrite (see dendrogram in Figure 11.2, bottom right and the histogram of path lengths in Figure 9.4, C1). The main metrical asymmetry between the basal and apical arborizations causes noticeable distinction between the more homogeneous bundle of basal profiles and the heterogeneous bundle family of the apical profiles (Figure 11.2, top right). At a given membrane conductivity $G_m = 40\,\mu S\,cm^{-2}$, the basal electrical profiles are gathered into a single, more or less homogeneous compact group (black arrow), whereas the apical path profiles significantly diverge and form three distinct bundles (open arrows). Within the apical arborization, asymmetrical subtrees are distinguished. In the main bifurcation located at about 450 μm from the soma, one sister branch is the origin of the most extended subtree 3. At 150 μm further from this point, another sister branch forms the next bifurcation from which two other subtrees emerge, the longer sub-tree 1 and shorter subtree 2. The distal parts of the longer sub-trees 3 and 1 are low efficiency with some preponderance of the subtree 1. The shortest subtree 2 is the most efficient in the passive current transfer. Hence, according to their transfer effectiveness the three apical subtrees are ordered in the sequence No. 2 > No. 1 > No. 3. The dendritic sites located at the same path distance from the soma on these asymmetrical subtrees differ significantly in their passive transfer effectiveness. However, within each subtree, one finds branches of similar effectiveness. An important observation is the critical difference in transfer effectiveness between the basal and apical parts of the reconstructed arborization.

These findings confirm the presence of more or less distinct bundles of electrical profiles in neurons with very different morphologies. The key words for explaining the presence of the bundles are *metrical asymmetry* and *branching complexity* of the dendritic paths.

11.1.2 Demonstration of cluster-type electrical structures

Although the observation of the bundles seems to be the rule for the tested neurons, how robust are they when different values of membrane conductivity are used in the computations? Are there alternatives to the bundle-type structure of the electrical path profiles? To answer this question, we perform a relevant type of mathematical analysis of electrical structures aimed at revealing robust groups with statistically significant within-group similarities and between-group differences in electrical transfer properties, the so-called *cluster analysis*.

Technique of cluster analysis

The cluster analysis of the electrical structures is performed using the k-means clustering method provided by CSS, STATISTICA (Statsoft, Tulsa, Oklahoma, USA, 1991). The corresponding algorithms are based on the theoretical derivations described in Hartigan (1975) and Zupan (1982). The cluster analysis is performed in a 2D parameter space in which each dendritic branch is described by two parameters of its steady electrical state: the mean voltage and the mean voltage gradient, i.e. the mean slope of the voltage decay in physical coordinates (Bras *et al.*, 1993; Korogod *et al.*, 1994). The mean voltage is computed as the sum of the voltages of isopotential compartments divided by the number of compartments of each branch. The mean gradient is computed as the voltage difference between the origin and the end of the branch, divided by branch length. The solution to the clustering problem, giving the number of clusters k, is obtained after a minimum of two iterations in all cases. The program starts with k random clusters and then moves objects (dendritic branches in our case) between these clusters, with the aim of: (1) minimizing the variability of the descriptive parameters (voltage and gradient) within the clusters and (2) maximizing the variability between the clusters. This is computationally equivalent to analysis of variance (ANOVA) in reverse, in the sense that the significance test in ANOVA evaluates the between-group variability against the within-group variability when computing the significance test for the hypothesis that the means of the groups are different from each other. Thus, in k-means clustering, the program moves the objects in and out of the clusters to get the most significant ANOVA results. For each cluster, in addition to its content with Euclidean distances of each member from the cluster centre in the parameter space, the program also provides computation of Euclidean distances to all other clusters, descriptive statistics (sample means and standard deviations) for every dimension, and analysis of within- and between-cluster variance (F tests of significance and P levels).

To apply this procedure to the electrical structures of the dendritic arborization of one abducens motoneuron (Figure 9.5, M5), first, the steady-state voltage along the dendritic branches is computed. Then, the mean voltage and gradient are computed as descriptive parameters for each dendritic branch. Finally, the cluster analysis is performed in the space of these two parameters for the set of all branches of the given motoneuron. As a result we know to which cluster each branch belongs. Each cluster is coded by its own colour, which is used to indicate the electrical profiles corresponding to all branches belonging to the given cluster. This is illustrated on the example of the arborization of the rat abducens motoneuron M5 in Figure 11.3. Dendritic branches that display similar voltages and gradients over a given distance constitute a cluster and are coloured in the same.

The number of clusters is found to be $k = 4$ in this case when computations are performed with $R_m = 3\,\text{k}\Omega \cdot \text{cm}^2$. Additional computations are made to test the dependency of the existence and the number of clusters on changes in the value of R_m. The number of clusters remains the same ($k = 4$) for computations with $R_m = 10\,\text{k}\Omega \cdot \text{cm}^2$ in both motoneurons. With $R_m = 1\,\text{k}\Omega \cdot \text{cm}^2$, the number of clusters increases to $k = 5$ resulting from the partition of cluster 2 into two sub-clusters (2a and 2b). The solution to the clustering problem is obtained after the minimum accepted number of two iterations with a statistically highly significant discrimination between all the clusters (see below). The clusters characterized by their mean values of voltages and gradients are sequentially ordered according to the somatofugal behaviour of these two parameters: from the highest mean voltages and gradients in cluster 1 to the lowest values in cluster 4 (see Table 1 in Korogod *et al.*, 1994 for details). To assess how distinct the clusters are, a statistical analysis is performed. Several quantitative estimates of discrimination between the clusters

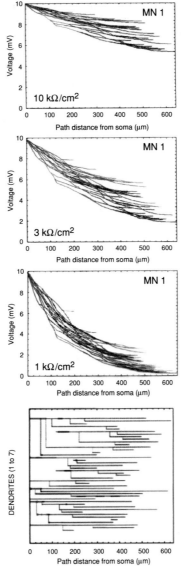

Figure 11.3 (Plate 2) Cluster-type electrical structure of reconstructed dendritic arborization of the abducens motoneuron shown in Figure 9.5 as cell M5. Three top boxes: The results of the cluster analysis of the somatofugal voltage decay are coded by colour and mapped on the profiles expressing the electrical structure of the M5 arborization, computed with $R_m = 1$, 3 and 10 k$\Omega \cdot$ cm^2. The steady voltage (ordinates) clamped to 10 mV above the rest potential at the soma decays along the branches with increasing path distance from the soma in μm (abscissae). Each branch ascribed to a cluster according to similarity of the mean voltage and gradient over a given distance is shown in the same colour. The mean voltages and gradients are the highest in cluster 1 (red) and lowest in cluster 4 (violet) and they are intermediate in clusters 2 (green) and 3 (cyan) containing the greatest numbers of profiles. Bottom box: The dendrogram of the arborization with the branches in the colours of the clusters that they belong to. (Rearranged from Korogod *et al.*, 1994.)

are computed. The magnitude of the F-test values obtained from the analysis of variance for each dimension (voltage and gradient) is an indication of how well the respective dimensions discriminate between the clusters. The results of ANOVA show that all values of F are $\gg 1$ and all significance levels but two are $\ll 0.001$, giving evidence of a highly significant discrimination between the clusters. This is true for the three values of R_m in this motoneuron (Table 2 in Korogod *et al.*, 1994). In the 'mean voltage-gradient' two-parameter space, Euclidean distances between the clusters and those between the branches within each cluster are computed to get quantitative estimates of the compactness of each cluster and the separation between them. The results of these computations (see Figure 3 and Table 3 in Korogod *et al.*, 1994) show that the mean Euclidean distances within the clusters are always several times smaller than those between the clusters for the three values of R_m, giving a further quantitative indication of good statistical discrimination between the clusters.

In Figure 11.3 with colour-coded cluster affiliation of the dendritic branches and of their electrical profiles, we notice an obvious correspondence between the colours and the bundles. Each bundle is mainly one colour, different bundles are different colours and the sequence of colours coding the clusters from higher to lower voltages and gradients corresponds to the sequence from upper to lower bundles. The colours indicate clusters and therefore the coloured bundles correspond to clusters of branches statistically discriminated according to their electrical transfer properties. The results of cluster analysis for the same arborization at different R_m are specially interesting. When R_m is changed from higher to lower values, the electrical structure evolves in a characteristic manner. At reduced $R_m = 1\,\mathrm{k\Omega} \cdot \mathrm{cm}^2$ (high conductance) the bundles of electrical profiles are compressed and visually less distinguished, reflecting a reduction of the difference between dendritic paths and branches in their transfer properties. However, the same recognizable bundles of profiles remain the same colours. This means that at the new lower level of transfer effectiveness, the within-group similarities and between-group differences remain statistically significant and the groups of electrical profiles remain statistically discriminated. This qualifies the observed electrical structures as the *cluster-type* structure.

There are more noteworthy details in the path profiles and dendrogram plots of the electrical clusters (Figure 11.3). First, the path distance location of branches belonging to different clusters. It is not surprising that cluster 1 (red, most efficient) and cluster 4 (violet, least efficient) are located, respectively, in the most proximal and most distal parts of the arborization. More interesting and even unexpected is that the branches belonging to the two other statistically distinct clusters 2 (green) and 3 (cyan) of intermediate effectiveness are located at approximately the same medium path distances from the soma. Second, almost all the individual dendrites contribute to both clusters 2 and 3 of intermediate effectiveness, which means similarity of their metrical asymmetry patterns. Third, the latter observation proves the possibility to use features of electrical structure, such as grouping the electrical profiles into bundles, as a detector of morphological parts of the arborization with similar metrical asymmetry. This is important because this morphological feature is not always obvious. Indeed, in the histogram of the distribution of the dendritic path length of the abducens motoneuron (Figure 9.5, M5), one can hardly distinguish clear modes of intermediate path lengths. Thanks to the electrical structure, one can thus detect rather obscure features of asymmetrical dendritic morphology.

11.2 Robustness of the electrical bundles

Simultaneous tonic activation of all synaptic inputs distributed over the whole arborization is the alternative to the activation of single-site inputs. Both types of activation are equally far from the physiological reality which lies in between these two extreme cases. The problem is that neither the number nor the exact locations of the activated synapses are known. However, one can assume that if certain geometry-induced features are present in both electrical structures computed for the two limiting, unrealistic cases, then these features are likely to be present in the 'intermediate' physiologically reasonable cases. Let's take such a feature as bundles of $T(x)$ profiles that correspond to the single-site activation case and ask the question whether such bundles are also formed by the voltage profiles representing the passive electrical structure of the same arborization, but receiving distributed inputs.

The electrical structure of the whole arborization with a passive membrane receiving homogeneously distributed synaptic activation represented by the family of voltage path profiles (Figure 11.4, b) is computed in the same way as in the case of an individual dendrite (Chapter 10). The family of voltage profiles forms almost a mirror image of the passive electrical structure represented by $T(x)$ profiles (Figure 11.4, a). The bundles of the electrical path profiles in (a), statistically characterized as clusters, have their 'mirror' bundles in the electrical structure of the same dendrites tonically activated via distributed inputs (b). We conclude that the robust geometry-induced feature present in both representations of the electrical structure are the bundles of the $T(x)$ and voltage path profiles. They indicate that, in the whole arborization, there are certain groups of branches and paths characterized by within-group similarities and between-group differences in processing of arbitrarily organized synaptic inputs for the same geometrical reasons.

Let us now perform one more test for the robustness of such geometry-induced electrical features of the whole arborization. We equip the dendritic membrane

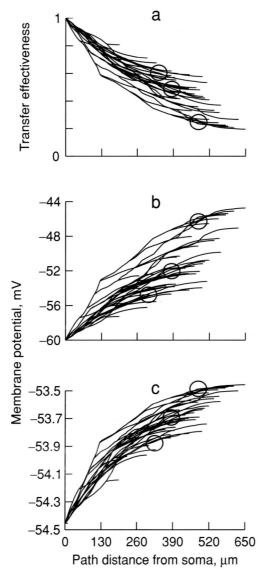

Figure 11.4 Electrical structures of the reconstructed dendritic arborization of abducens motoneuron (cell M5 in Figure 9.5) with passive (a, b) and active, Hodgkin–Huxley type (c) properties of the dendritic membrane. Electrical structures are represented by the path profiles of the relative effectiveness of the somatopetal current transfer $T(x)$ from single-site sources in passive dendrites (a) and by the path profiles of the membrane potentials (b, c) resulting from tonic activation of excitatory synaptic inputs homogeneously distributed over the dendrites with passive (b) or active (c) membranes. (Rearranged from Korogod *et al.*, 1998.)

with voltage-dependent conductances of the Hodgkin–Huxley type and submit the dendritic arborization to the same type of distributed tonic synaptic activation as in the preceding case for passive dendrites. In the case of individual dendrites, although there is an asymmetry-induced divergence of the voltage path profiles (Figure 10.3, E), due to the currents through the voltage-dependent extra-synaptic conductances, the profiles diverge less than in the case when this dendrite has a passive extra-synaptic membrane (Figure 10.3, A). Since such non-linearity of the dendritic membrane erodes the asymmetry-induced electrical effects, can it also erode the asymmetry-induced grouping of the dendritic branches and paths?

Consider the family of path profiles of the membrane voltages generated by the same dendritic arborization with an active (Hodgkin–Huxley type) membrane in response to tonic activation of distributed synaptic inputs that provides another active type of electrical structure (Figure 11.4, c). This type looks also like a mirror image, though somewhat deformed, of the passive structure (a) with still recognizable distinct 'mirror' bundles. Hence, the presence of bundles corresponding to the groups of branches in similar electrical states is a common feature induced by the dendritic geometry, namely by multiple elements with similar metrical asymmetry.

11.3 Dynamic reconfigurations of the whole electrical structure

How are the general properties of activity-dependent reconfiguration of the passive electrical structure found in individual dendrites (Chapter 10) manifested in whole arborizations of different types?

11.3.1 The size effect

We will take specific examples of complex arborizations that highlight the effects of such structural features as the size and metrical asymmetry patterns. Among our library neurons, the greatest difference in the overall size of the dendritic arborizations (more than four times) is found between the cerebellar Purkinje cells and neocortical layer 5 pyramidal cells. There is approximately the same difference between basal and apical dendrites of the same pyramidal neuron. These neuron types are worth considering in this context because they also have a special pattern of metrical asymmetry which induces a noticeable feature of the passive electrical structure: the bundles of the passive electrical profiles.

We can compute the passive transfer ratio $T(x)$ for the Purkinje neuron P1 (Figure 9.3) and the pyramidal neuron C1 (Figure 9.4) at different values of the membrane conductivity G_m, and select plots with similar maximum divergence of the electrical path profiles. These data are shown in Figure 11.5.

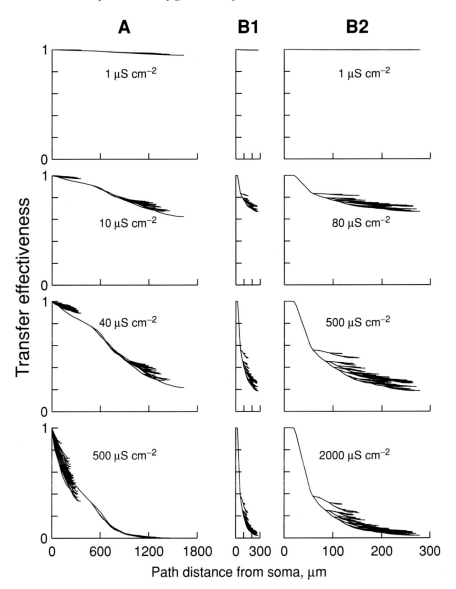

Figure 11.5 Size dependence of dynamic reconfiguration of the electrical structures of neocortical layer 5 pyramidal neuron (A) and Purkinje neuron (B1 and B2). The current transfer effectiveness $T(x)$ (ordinate, dimensionless) is computed as a function of the path distance from the soma (abscissae, μm) along all the dendritic paths of the arborization at different values of the membrane conductivity G_m indicated in μS cm^{-2} on the corresponding plot.

At low G_m values, e.g. $1 \ \mu S \ cm^{-2}$, the electrical profiles of each arborization merge into a single bundle at a level close to the maximal relative transfer effectiveness $T(x) = 1$. In both neurons, an increase in the membrane conductivity G_m (decrease of the membrane resistivity $R_m = 1/G_m$) leads to the segregation of electrical profiles that neatly correspond to asymmetrical subtrees. In the pyramidal neuron, at $G_m = 10 \ \mu S \ cm^{-2}$, the bundles of electrical profiles in the apical sub-trees are clearly segregated, whereas those in the basal dendrites remain essentially merged at a high effectiveness level. At the same G_m value, the electrical profiles of the whole arborization of the Purkinje neuron also remain essentially merged. To get approximately the same segregation as that obtained at $10 \ \mu S \ cm^{-2}$ for the pyramidal neuron, the membrane conductivity of the Purkinje dendrites has to be increased almost by an order of magnitude, up to $80 \ \mu S \ cm^{-2}$. The maximum segregation of the electrical profiles of the apical arborization in the pyramidal neuron is observed at $G_m = 40 \ \mu S \ cm^{-2}$ and that of the whole arborization of the Purkinje neuron at $500 \ \mu S \ cm^{-2}$, that is 12 times greater. In the pyramidal neuron, at $G_m = 500 \ \mu S \ cm^{-2}$, the apical electrical profiles are again virtually merged, but at a low level close to 0, whereas the profiles corresponding to the basal dendrites are separated almost maximally. Increase of G_m up to $2000 \ \mu S \ cm^{-2}$ in the Purkinje neuron reduces the segregation of the electrical profiles, which approach the low level.

The results show that, in both neurons, it is possible to define three characteristic ranges of membrane conductivity: *the low-conductance range*, in which all the electrical profiles are closely adjacent to each other at a level of relatively high transfer effectiveness; *the high-conductance range*, in which the electrical profiles are also closely adjacent, but at a level of relatively low relative effectiveness; *the medium-conductance range*, in which the profiles corresponding to asymmetrical subtrees are maximally segregated. The limits of these ranges are shifted to greater values, approximately by one order of magnitude, in Purkinje neurons compared to pyramidal neurons. The same is true for the range limits corresponding to the basal dendrites compared to apical dendrites in the pyramidal neuron arborization.

An important question arises from the observation of compressed electrical profiles at very low and very high values of membrane conductivity. As in these cases, all the profiles merge into a very narrow single bundle, it seems like the metrical asymmetry becomes unimportant and the grouping of the dendritic branches and paths does not exist anymore. To check whether this is true or not, we can expand the scale along the $T(x)$ axis so that the visual difference between top and bottom profiles increases approximately to the same extent as in the case of intermediate membrane conductances. The outcome is shown in Figure 11.6 for the dendritic arborization of the Purkinje neuron. In the reference plots of $T(x)$ in full scale from

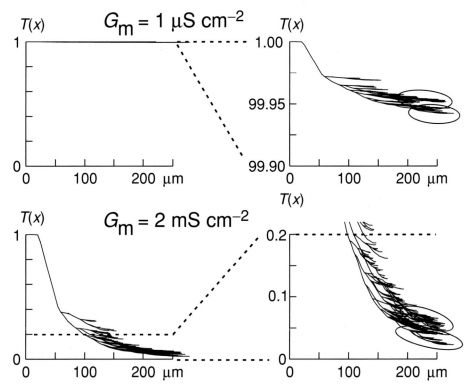

Figure 11.6 Robustness of the asymmetry-induced grouping of the dendritic branches and paths according to similarity and dissimilarity of their passive transfer properties. The families of the passive electrical profiles $T(x)$ computed at the membrane conductivities $G_m = 1$ μS cm^{-2} and 2 mS cm^{-2} (indicated above the corresponding plots) and shown in the same full scale as in Figure 11.5 (left) and expanded (right).

0 to 1 (left), one cannot see the bundles, at least the three which were distinct at intermediate conductivities (cf. Figure 11.5, A). All the profiles are compressed into a narrow single bundle at very low conductivity (1 μS cm^{-2}, top) into a dense strip at high conductivity (2 mS cm^{-2}, bottom). However, when the same $T(x)$ profiles are plotted with an expanded ordinate scale (right), one sees the groups of the profiles (enveloped by ellipses) which correspond to those observed in Figure 11.5, A, e.g. at $G_m = 500$ μS cm^{-2} and even 80 μS cm^{-2}. Hence, although the difference in the passive transfer effectiveness between the asymmetrical paths becomes small at very low and high membrane conductivities, the general 'cluster-type' features of the electrical structure are conserved. For the groups of asymmetrical branches and paths, the between-group differences and the within-group electrical similarities remain.

11.4 Spatial aspects of reconfigured electrical structure

Considering the asymmetry-induced divergence of the passive electrical path profiles of the whole arborizations at different membrane conductivities, we focused
in the previous section on the width of the strip of profiles in the dimension along
the ordinate $T(x)$. Here we focus on another dimension and consider the width
of the same strip along the abscissa, i.e. the path distance from the soma. This
width can be considered at different levels of transfer effectiveness $T(x)$. From
this we know how far the proximal dendritic path section extends, in which the
transfer effectiveness exceeds a given level. This aspect of the dynamic reconfiguration of electrical structures we consider for different types of motoneurons.
The selected digitized motoneurons (Figure 9.5) have different sizes, from small
(spinal motoneuron M3 of young rat) to medium (rat abducens motoneuron M4)
and large spinal motoneurons (cat M1 and frog M2). When the reconfigurations
of the electrical structures of the pyramidal and Purkinje neurons were compared
(Figure 11.5) we took different values of G_m that provide similar divergence of
electrical profiles. Now we explore the difference in $T(x)$ profiles computed for
four motoneurons in the same conditions: each at three different $G_m = 0.01, 0.1$
and 1.0 mS cm^{-2} that correspond to the membrane resistivity values $R_m = 100, 10$
and 1 k$\Omega \cdot$ cm^2 (Figure 11.7).

Let us consider four aspects of the same plots. First, like in the similar plots
for Purkinje and pyramidal neurons, we consider in general the compactness of
the whole family of path profiles at different values of membrane resistivity. For
that we compare how far from each other the profiles along the $T(x)$ ordinate are.
Second, we note in which range of transfer effectiveness the profiles fall. For that
we use $T(x) = 0.5$ as the reference level and distinguish only two ranges: high,
with $T(x) > 0.5$ and low, with $T(x) < 0.5$. Third, we note at which path distances
x the $T(x)$ profiles cross the reference 0.5 level and from x coordinates of these
cross-points we infer the path distance extent of the highly effective dendritic
domain. Fourth, ultimately we specially note the distance between the right-most
and left-most cross-points, which can be considered as an indicator of the metrical
asymmetry of the electrically high-efficiency sections of the asymmetrical dendritic
paths.

Consider the first aspect and make sure that, in the reconstructed motoneurons, the size-dependence of the divergence of the electrical path profiles corresponds to that observed in the arborizations of Purkinje and pyramidal neurons. In
each motoneuron, the $T(x)$ profiles are most compact at the highest tested $R_m = 100$ k$\Omega \cdot$ cm^2 and diverge at intermediate $R_m = 10$ k$\Omega \cdot$ cm^2 (Figure 11.7, black and
dark grey lines). In some cases, the family splits into distinct bundles having spe-
cific features in each arborization. At the lowest $R_m = 1$ k$\Omega \cdot$ cm^2 the profiles (light

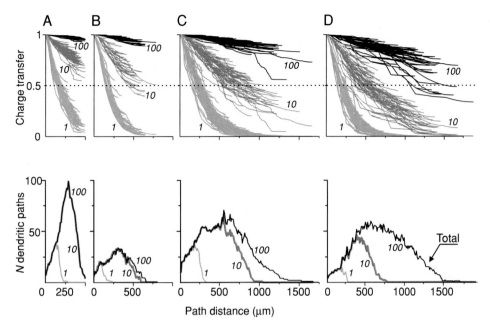

Figure 11.7 Passive electrical structures and their reconfiguration induced by changes in the membrane resistivity R_m for the dendritic arborizations of four motoneurons shown in Figure 9.5: rat spinal (A), rat abducens (B), cat (C) and frog (D) spinal motoneurons. Top: Electrical structures are represented by the path profiles of the somatopetal charge transfer effectiveness (ordinates) as a function of the path distance from soma (abscissae) computed for $R_m = 100\,\text{k}\Omega \cdot \text{cm}^2$ (black lines), $10\,\text{k}\Omega \cdot \text{cm}^2$ (dark grey lines) and $1\,\text{k}\Omega \cdot \text{cm}^2$ (light grey lines). The profiles above and below the dotted line at $T(x) = 0.5$ correspond to the low-efficiency $(T(x) < 0.5)$ and high-efficiency $(T(x) > 0.5)$ domains of the dendritic paths. The path coordinates of the cross-points of profiles on the $T(x) = 0.5$ line define the path distance from the soma to the border of the high-efficiency domain. Bottom: The complexity function of the arborizations and their high-efficiency domains represented by the number of the dendritic path profiles (ordinates) with $T(x) = 0.5$ at three values of R_m: $100\,\text{k}\Omega \cdot \text{cm}^2$ (black line), $10\,\text{k}\Omega \cdot \text{cm}^2$ (dark grey line) and $1\,\text{k}\Omega \cdot \text{cm}^2$ (light grey line), as a function of the path distance from soma (abscissae). The number of profiles is equal to the number of dendritic paths. At $R_m = 100\,\text{k}\Omega \cdot \text{cm}^2$, the entire arborizations are in the high-efficiency domain of the motoneurons (A–C) with only one exception (D). Their complexity function is superimposed on that of the entire arborizations (black lines). In D, the two functions display a slight difference (Total). (From Korogod et al., 2000.)

grey lines) of the shortest arborization (A, rat spinal motoneuron) further diverge, whereas those of the larger motoneurons (B–D) become compressed again, especially in the distal parts of the largest cat (C) and frog (D) motoneurons, where they overlap at nearly zero level. Hence, in this respect the reconfiguration of the electrical structures caused by changes in R_m in small and large motoneurons is in good correspondence with that observed in the arborizations of Purkinje and pyramidal neurons.

Now consider the second and third aspects of the reconfiguration picture. The partition of the arborizations into two arbitrary domains of charge transfer effectiveness (low and high efficiency) reveals that three of the four motoneurons have their whole arborization in the high-efficiency domain under $R_m = 100 \text{ k}\Omega \cdot \text{cm}^2$. The bundles of the shortest dendritic arborization (Figure 11.7, A) are the most compressed up to the distal tips, with values of $T(x)$ between 0.95 and 1.0, indicating a close similarity of all the dendritic paths in their transfer effectiveness. The behaviour of the rat abducens (Figure 11.7, B) and the cat motoneuron (Figure 11.7, C) is similar under $R_m = 100 \text{ k}\Omega \cdot \text{cm}^2$, except for the longest path distances, in which a slight tendency toward decompression is observed in the cat. In the frog motoneuron (Figure 11.7, D), the electrical profiles are more decompressed even at $R_m = 100 \text{ k}\Omega \cdot \text{cm}^2$, with some of the longest profiles in the low-efficiency domain. At $R_m = 10 \text{ k}\Omega \cdot \text{cm}^2$, all arborizations are decompressed, showing a much wider variation in the charge transfer effectiveness of the paths. Except for the rat spinal motoneuron, the longest profiles fall into the low-efficiency domain beyond 400–500 μm from the soma, some of them even reaching values close to zero efficiency at 1500 μm from the soma in the frog motoneuron (Figure 11.7, D). Because the rat spinal motoneuron (Figure 11.7, A) has no dendritic paths longer than 500 μm, all the profiles remain in the high-efficiency domain although they are very decompressed in their distal parts with $T(x)$ in the range between 0.93 and 0.56. Under $R_m = 1 \text{ k}\Omega \cdot \text{cm}^2$, a dramatic reduction in the high-efficiency domain characterizes all arborizations. The bundles of profiles are compressed again in the four arborizations and the $T(x)$ profiles decay abruptly over the first 250 μm from the soma to reach the low-efficiency domain. The longest path profiles of the cat and frog motoneurons fall to values close to zero efficiency between 550 and 700 μm from the soma, whereas none of the profiles of rat spinal or abducens motoneurons reach zero $T(x)$, even in their most distal parts.

Ultimately, consider the fourth aspect of the reconfiguration picture: the dispersion of the borders of the highly effective proximal parts of the dendritic paths estimated by the width of the cross-section of the family of electrical profiles by the reference level line $T(x) = 0.5$. A noteworthy feature is observed in the profiles for cat and frog motoneurons at medium and low R_m: with change of R_m from 10 to 1 $\text{k}\Omega \cdot \text{cm}^2$ the cross-points shift to the left and become closer to each other (the left-shifted cross-sections are narrower). This means that, in terms of the path distances, the high-efficiency domains of the dendritic arborizations become smaller and less asymmetrical when R_m is reduced. Another noteworthy feature is seen when comparing the path distance location of the cross-sections of the electrical profiles of different motoneurons. When R_m is reduced to 1 $\text{k}\Omega \cdot \text{cm}^2$

the shorter cross-sections of small and large arborizations are located at about the same 250 μm path distances from the soma. This means decreasing differences between small and large arborizations in the path distance extent of their highly effective domains.

11.5 Complexity of the whole arborization and its electrical domains

The reconfiguration of the electrical structures of the whole arborizations of four motoneurons caused by introducing different values of R_m reveals an unequal reduction in the their high-efficiency domains. It also indicates clear quantitative differences between the sensitivity of $T(x)$ of each arborization to changes in R_m. The representation of the global electrical structure in physical coordinates provides a direct estimate of the proportion of the path extent in the high-efficiency domain, but the number of paths in this domain often is not resolved because of the overlapping of electrical profiles in narrow bundles. To solve this problem, we use the fact that the dendritic subtrees and their corresponding bundles of electrical profiles are homeomorphous (topologically equivalent). Here we use the complexity function introduced by Korogod *et al.* (2000) to describe the composition of the dendritic domains of high efficiency. The complexity of any dendritic domain is defined by the number of dendritic paths as a function of the path distance from the soma. At zero path distance, the complexity function is equal to the number of primary dendrites emerging from the soma. As the path distance increases, the number of paths increases by 1 when a bifurcation occurs or decrements by 1 when a path terminates. The complexity function increases in the spatial domain where the branchings prevail over terminals and decreases where the terminals prevail. It is used to further characterize the number of dendritic paths included in the high-efficiency domain under the three values of R_m (Figure 11.7, bottom). The surface areas below the plots of the complexity function show the total length of the dendritic paths in the domain. For $R_m = 100 \, k\Omega \cdot cm^2$, the entire arborizations are highly effective in all motoneurons but one. Correspondingly, the complexity function is the same for the whole arborization and the high-efficiency domain (Figure 11.7, black lines). The exception is the frog motoneuron, in which a small difference is observed (Figure 11.7, D, black line and line marked Total). In the rat spinal motoneuron, with path lengths that do not exceed 480 μm, the maximum complexity (99 paths) occurs at the shortest path distance of 280 μm (Figure 11.7, A). For the rat abducens motoneuron with a dendritic extension of 770 μm, the maximum complexity is smaller (35 paths) and occurs at 346 μm from the soma (Figure 11.7, B). In the cat spinal motoneuron, the maximum complexity (70 paths) occurs at about 540 μm, whereas the longest path is 1627 μm (Figure 11.7, C). In the frog spinal motoneuron, the maximum complexity (60 paths) is at 470 μm from the soma, and the arborization extends up to 1824 μm (Figure 11.7, D). The reduction in R_m to 10 kΩ/cm^2 has no effect on the complexity function of the high-efficiency domain in the rat spinal motoneuron, whereas the function decreases by approximately 5%, 20% and 60% in the other three motoneurons. In the two small motoneurons, the same changes in R_m introduced almost no changes in the complexity of their high-efficiency domains. However, a further reduction in R_m (1 kΩ/cm^2) induces large changes in both path extent and complexity function in the four motoneurons. The complexity function ascertains that the high-efficiency domain can be reduced to a small number of dendritic branches efficiently connected to the soma under low values of R_m. We conclude that the complexity function gives additional quantitative information that is not retrieved from observation of the electrical profiles.

For neurobiologists, the electrical structures of the whole arborizations represented by families of curves remain a rather unusual abstract object although they contain extremely rich information for understanding the electrical properties of dendritic arborizations. Our fine analysis of dendritic profiles by explaining the biophysical mechanisms that rule their electrical structures provides the necessary and fundamental principles on which we can now rely to proceed to the exploration of the 3D shapes of the biological neuron.

References

Bras, H., Korogod, S., Driencourt, Y., Gogan, P. and Tyč-Dumont, S. (1993). Stochastic geometry and electrotonic architecture of dendritic arborization of a brain-stem motoneuron. *Eur. J. Neurosci.*, **5**:1405–1493.

Hartigan, J. A. (1975). *Clustering Algorithms*, New York: John Wiley & Sons, Inc.

Korogod, S. M., Bras, H., Sarana, V. N., Gogan, P. and Tyč-Dumont, S. (1994). Electrotonic clusters in the dendritic arborisation of abducens motoneurons in the rat. *Eur. J. Neurosci.*, **6**:1517–1527.

Korogod, S. M., Kulagina, I. B., Horcholle-Bossavit, G., Gogan, P. and Tyč-Dumont, S. (2000). Activity-dependent reconfiguration of the effective dendritic field of motoneurons. *J. Comp. Neurol.*, **422**:18–34.

Korogod, S. M., Kulagina, I. B. and Tyč-Dumont, S. (1998). Transfer properties of neuronal dendrites with tonically activated conductances. *Neurophysiology*, **30**:203–207.

Zupan, J. (1982). *Clustering of Large Data Sets*, New York: Research Studies Press.

12

Electrical structures in 3D dendritic space

For the biologist, the gap between results of model computation and live neurons is filled when an electrical structure is mapped on the static anatomy of the dendritic field of neurons. The speaking likeness of these 3D images opens a new way of thinking by providing a functional image of 3D dendritic space. Indeed it is new because the question of the electrical state of the whole dendritic space is rarely addressed, although critical for understanding how the neuron processes its inputs.

The three types of neurons investigated here have their own idiosyncratic 3D dendritic pattern so well described in morphological words. In Chapters 10 and 11, we explore the arborizations as determinants of their spatial electrical properties without referring to the dendritic geometry as an object inserted in physical 3D space. The restriction of this view can be explained with a simple analogy. This is a view of the dendrites 'from the inside'.

We can imagine the dendritic arborization as a 'cave maze' in the brain's depths. When we are inside the maze, we do not perceive its 3D shape. We can wander inside, uncoiling 'Ariadne's thread' on our path from the entry (the soma) to the deadlocks (the distal tips) and then measure the length of the threads between those points to find the path lengths. Another spatial information available from the interior view is the diameter of the 'cave' at each site along the path. Knowing the lengths and diameters of all the paths in such a labyrinth is sufficient for computing the spatial electrical structures. So, the arborization as the determinant of the spatial electrical properties can be exhaustively characterized. Now, we escape from the dendritic maze and look at it 'from outside'. From the exterior viewpoint, we can observe the geography of dendritic space, we search for elements of dendritic arborization bearing similar or dissimilar electrical properties and define where in the 3D space these elements are located. This is necessary for answering further the question of how the dendrites process synaptic inputs delivered in the 3D space of the brain where the arborizations are inserted.

Let us go to the 3D dendritic space of the neurons in our library and see the 3D arrangement of their electrical maps which were described from the 'interior viewpoint' in the preceding chapters.

12.1 The 3D electrical structures of Purkinje neurons

We start with the electrical maps of the dendritic space of Purkinje neurons. This space has the most advantageous geography: it is planar and the dendritic elements are located very close to each other, which facilitates greatly the comparison of their electrical states.

Figure 12.1 shows the electrical structures of the reconstructed planar dendritic arborizations of six Purkinje neurons (Kulagina *et al.*, 2007). Each electrical structure is represented by a dendritic map of steady voltage that is identical to the map of passive transfer profiles $T(x)$ (see Chapter 6). The comparison of the six electrical structures (plots P1 to P6 in Figure 12.1) reveals common and cell-specific features. The common feature is the organization of the path profiles into more or less dense bundles corresponding to sets of paths with similar voltage transfer. The voltage profiles corresponding to the asymmetrical dendritic paths are separated, although they run along side each other over path distances of several tens of micrometres. In all cells, they indicate the presence of multiple segments situated at equidistance from the soma, characterized by different voltages and thus different passive transfer properties.

The cell-specific features are represented by different deviations of the voltages at the distal dendritic tips from the same reference voltage ($-60\,\mathrm{mV}$) at the soma. These dendritic voltages range from about $-66.5\,\mathrm{mV}$ in P5 to $-68.5\,\mathrm{mV}$ in P2. The voltage difference between the tips of the shortest and longest dendritic paths range from about $3.5\,\mathrm{mV}$ in P1 to about $6\,\mathrm{mV}$ in P3, P4 and P6. Finally, the number and mutual position of individual path profiles and their pattern itself are cell-specific. On the 3D images of the arborizations (Figure 12.1), dendritic domains with similar (same colour) or dissimilar (different colours) voltages are situated in dendritic fields. We find two main types of partition of the dendritic arborizations according to spatial transfer properties. In four cells (P1, P3, P4 and P6), the domains look like planar sectors approximately limited by radii (dashed lines) emerging from major branching points. In each case, one can distinguish sectors of low (L), medium (M) and high (H) effectiveness. Noteworthy, in four cases, the electrical structure is clearly partitioned into radial sectors according to transfer properties. Therefore we conclude that a *sector-like* arrangement of the electrical structure is typical for planar dendritic arborizations of Purkinje neurons, at least for this small sample. The identified sectors of low, medium and high transfer effectiveness are spatially

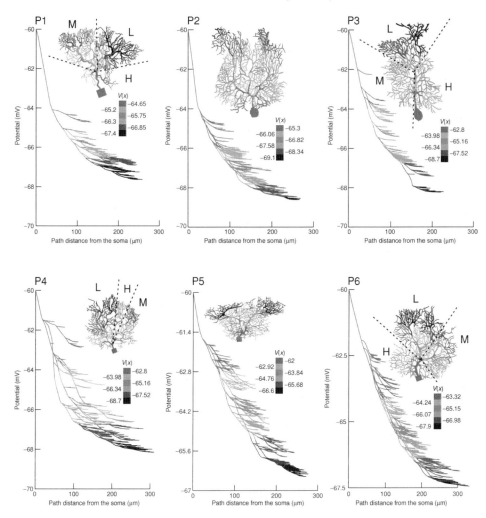

Figure 12.1 (Plate 3) Electrical sectors in the reconstructed planar dendritic fields of Purkinje neurons P1 to P6 (Figure 9.3). For each cell, the passive membrane voltages (ordinates, mV) are computed along the dendrites as a function of the path distance x from the soma (abscissae, μm), colour-coded with the six-colour palettes (inserts) and mapped on the plot of electrical profiles and 3D image of the arborization. Same or different colours indicate dendritic domains with similar or dissimilar voltages (passive transfer properties). In each case, the domains of low (L), medium (M) and high (H) depolarization/effectiveness are identified. In P1, P3, P4 and P6 the domains look like planar sectors approximately limited by radii (dashed lines) emerging from major branching points. In P2 and P5, the partition of the dendritic fields appears more patchy. (From Kulagina *et al.*, 2007.)

separated and ordered by the polar angle indicating polar angular arrangement of the branching asymmetry.

12.2 The 3D electrical structure of pyramidal neurons

The dendritic space of the cortical pyramidal neurons is far more complex. The pattern of stratification of all cortical regions displays a common architectural prin-ciple of vertical and horizontal orientation of its structural elements, being present in the most simple as well as the most complicated kinds of cortex. The unique shape of the dendritic apparatus of the pyramidal neuron adheres to this principle. The singularity of the electrical structure of the pyramidal neuron arborization lies in a similar type of stratification which we classify as layered (Figure 12.2).

The 3D map of its passive transfer effectiveness (Figure 12.2) shows that the apical dendrite transfers the signals arriving at the main stem segments in layers 4–2 with differing effectiveness. The electrical structure of the apical tuft composed of tangential branches to the cortex surface has the spatial arrangement of the sector-field or sector-like type, common to the other types of neurons already described. For instance, the right sector of the tuft tangential field is occupied by the apical subtree 3, composed of the longest and electrically least efficient branches (Figure 12.2), whereas the right sector is formed by more efficient tuft branches of the subtree 2. The 3D space of the basal arborization in layer 5 is filled with the most proximal and efficient branches.

12.3 The 3D electrical structures of motoneurons

The arborization of the motoneurons is a true 3D structure as the dendrites radiate in all directions in the 3D space around the soma. Each individual dendrite occupies its own spatial sector in 3D space and the spatial sectors of different dendrites do not intersect (Bras *et al.*, 1987, 1993; Korogod *et al.*, 1994). We know that the presence of clusters is demonstrated in the electrical structure of the two abducens motoneurons shown in Figure 11.3 (Korogod *et al.*, 1994).

The mapping of these clusters on their 3D images in Figure 12.3 reveals their specific features. With no surprise we find that the branches belonging to the most effective cluster 1 occupy the region of 3D space that is the most proximal to the soma (coloured red in Figure 12.3). Also not surprising is the location of the least efficient cluster 4 members on the far periphery of the 3D dendritic space. Noteworthy is the location of the branches forming clusters 2 and 3, characterized by intermediate values of the somatopetal current transfer effectiveness as esti-mated by the mean values of the somatofugal voltage and voltage gradient. On the dendrogram plot (Figure 11.3), one can see the branches of the same dendrite

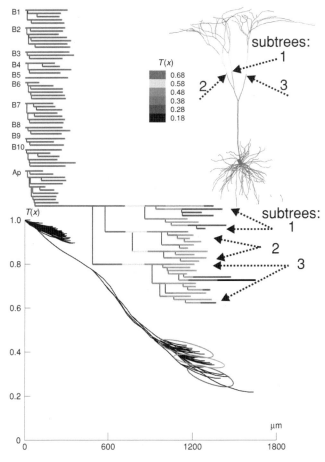

Figure 12.2 (Plate 4) Passive electrical structure of reconstructed dendritic arborizations of the pyramidal neuron (cell C1) of layer 5 of the neocortex. Bottom: Path profiles of the relative effectiveness of the somatopetal current transfer $T(x)$ (ordinate, dimensionless; abscissa, path distance from the soma, μm). Top left and right: Respectively, the dendrogram and 3D image of the reconstructed arborization, on which the colour-coded values of $T(x)$ are mapped (the six-colour palette is shown in the insert). B1–B10: basal dendrites. Ap: apical dendrites with several relatively short oblique dendrites. Arrows 1–3 indicate three main apical subtrees. Ellipses envelope groups of the path profiles corresponding to the dendritic branches with relatively high (green), medium (blue) and low (magenta) transfer effectiveness.

located at similar path distances from the soma, but belonging to different clusters according to their transfer properties in the intermediate ranges (clusters 2 and 3). In 3D space (Figure 12.3), these cluster 2 and 3 branches occur at similar air-way distances from the soma at the same spatial angle, which is the 3D domain occupied by the given individual dendrite. Hence, the branches with intermediate, but

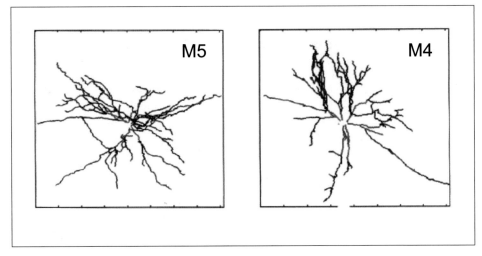

Figure 12.3 (Plate 5) 3D location of electrical clusters of the dendritic arborization of abducens motoneurons. (From Korogod *et al.*, 1994.)

significantly discriminated transfer effectiveness share the same sectors of the 3D space of the arborization. This occurs in different spatial angles around the soma. Such an arrangement of transfer properties in 3D space can by qualified as the electrical structure of the *shared-sector* type. In dendritic arborizations with such electrical structures, the dendrites occupying different spatial sectors of the peri-somatic 3D space transfer currents from synaptic inputs to these sectors with significantly discriminated levels of effectiveness. This looks like coarse (low effectiveness) and fine (high effectiveness) tuning of the dendritic signal receiver serving the given spatial sector of the 3D dendritic field.

12.4 High-efficiency domain of the motoneuronal arborizations in 3D

To finish with the passive electrical structures, let's consider now the dynamic reconfiguration of high- and low-efficiency domains in the 3D space of dendritic arborizations with the example of a large and a small motoneuron (cells M1 and M3 in Figure 9.5). The data obtained from Figure 11.7 are mapped onto the 3D images of the arborizations (Figure 12.4) (Korogod *et al.*, 2000).

At high $R_m = 100\,\text{k}\Omega \cdot \text{cm}^2$, the entire projection fields are in the high-efficiency domain, whereas the number of dendritic branches efficiently connected to the soma is decreased dramatically at low $R_m = 1\,\text{k}\Omega \cdot \text{cm}^2$. The effective zone is reduced to a small sphere around the soma in both large and small motoneurons. At intermediate $R_m = 10\,\text{k}\Omega \cdot \text{cm}^2$, the large motoneuron with long dendritic paths has many distal branches in the low-efficiency domain compared to the small motoneuron. The

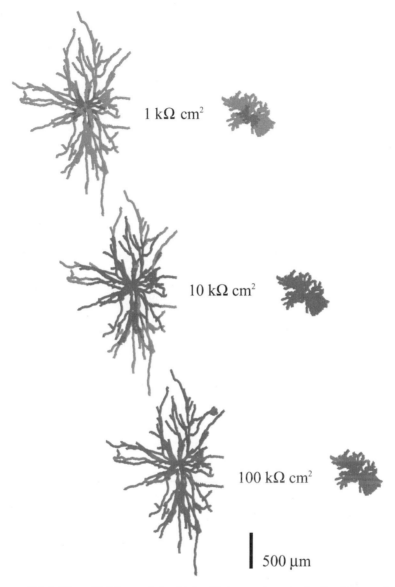

Figure 12.4 (Plate 6) Maps of the high-efficiency domain (red) of cat and rat spinal motoneurons (respectively M1 and M3 of Figure 9.5) for three values of R_{m}. At $R_{\mathrm{m}} = 100\,\mathrm{k\Omega \cdot cm^2}$, the dendritic fields of both arborizations are in the high-efficiency domain, with a similar weight for all synaptic inputs. By reducing the value of R_{m}, the high-efficiency domains shrink and many dendritic branches are disconnected functionally from the soma. (From Korogod *et al.*, 2000.)

larger the dendritic field, the greater is the variability of the 3D extent of the high-efficiency domain. The long dendritic paths of the cat motoneuron display a higher sensitivity to reduction in the values of R_m, while short dendritic paths of the rat motoneurons are only affected by values of $R_m < 10 \text{ k}\Omega \cdot \text{cm}^2$. The size-dependence of the reconfiguration of the electrical structure demonstrated in Chapter 9 is verified here for the 3D structure.

12.5 Bistable dendritic field

We know that electrical bistability is provided by an N-shaped I–V relation for the dendritic membrane due to the presence of non-linear synaptic conductances. This configuration is the most probable in live neurons that are embedded in numerous networks and involved in different functional activities. According to background activity, the neuron modifies the dynamics of its dendritic state to dwell in perfect harmony with the demand of the current operations performed by the neuronal networks. This electrical behaviour is well demonstrated by computing the current density in the dendrites in two stable states.

12.5.1 Maps of current density

Simulations (Korogod *et al.*, 2002) performed on the abducens motoneuron M4 are illustrated in Figure 9.5. In this motoneuron, the electrical bistability is provided by an N-shaped I–V relation for the dendritic membrane due to the presence of non-linear NMDA-type glutamatergic synaptic conductances. The protocol is the same as for individual dendrites with distributed NMDA-type synaptic inputs (Chapter 10). When the whole dendritic arborization of this motoneuron is tonically activated by homogeneously distributed NMDA synaptic inputs with two values of synaptic conductances fixed just below ($\overline{G}_{NMDA} = 3.3 \text{ mS cm}^{-2}$) and above ($\overline{G}_{NMDA} = 3.4 \text{ mS cm}^{-2}$) the upper limit of bistability, the current density is unevenly distributed over the arborization. This is clearly demonstrated in Figure 12.5, where the current density computed in the low (A and C) and high (B and D) depolarization states (*downstate* and *upstate*, respectively) is mapped onto the 3D image (A and B) and the dendrogram (C and D) of the arborization.

In the *downstate*, the dendritic field displays a ring of small current density (-0.33 nA cm^{-2}) around the soma with an irregular outline depending on the dendritic paths. The remaining part of the arborization shows only small differences in current density, with three exceptions found in the most complex asymmetrical dendrites 3 and 5 (Figure 12.5, C) and in the very distal tip of dendrite 2, with a high current density of -0.43 nA cm^{-2}. The dendritic fields of each of these three dendrites are spatially well separated, projecting in three different regions.

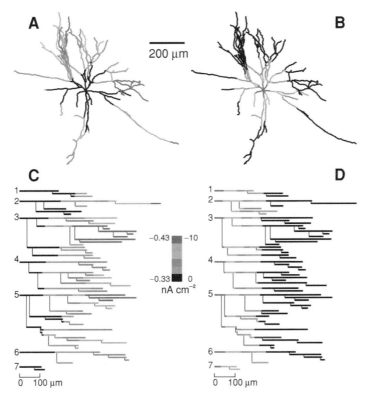

Figure 12.5 (Plate 7) Bistable spatial distributions of the total membrane current density mapped on the dendritic arborization of motoneuron M4 shown in Figure 9.5. A: Snapshot of the plane projection of 3D reconstructed arborization and C: the corresponding dendrogram at downstate with $\overline{G}_{NMDA} = 3.3$ mS cm^{-2}, just below the limit of the range of electrical bistability. B: Snapshot of the plane projection of 3D arborization and D: the corresponding dendrogram at the upstate with $\overline{G}_{NMDA} = 3.4$ mS cm^{-2}, just above the upper limit of the range of electrical bistability. The computed current density is colour-coded and scaled in six equal steps from -0.33 to -0.43 nA cm^{-2} for A and C and from 0 to -10 nA cm^{-2} for B and D. (From Korogod *et al.*, 2002.)

Noteworthy, the inward current of greatest density is generated in the distal branches of the most complex dendrites 3 and 5, which are the branches placed in the least efficient cluster 4 according to their passive membrane properties (cf. right box in Figure 12.3). Comparison of the same figures shows that many branches being at the same path distances from the soma, generate noticeably different inward currents that also correspond to their affiliation with different clusters.

In the *upstate*, the current density maps are totally inverted. The most proximal dendritic branches generate high current density up to -10 nA cm^{-2} over the first 80 μm from the soma. Past the first 200–250 μm from the soma, the current

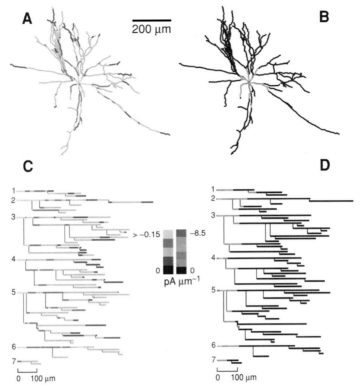

Figure 12.6 (Plate 8) Bistable spatial distribution of the current transfer effectiveness mapped on the same dendritic arborization as shown in Figure 12.5. A: Snapshot of the 3D reconstructed arborization and C: the dendrogram in the downstate. B: Snapshot of the 3D arborization and D: the dendrogram in the upstate. The computed core current increments are colour-coded and scaled in six equal steps from 0 to $-0.15\,\mathrm{pA\,\mu m^{-1}}$ for A and C and from 0 to $-8.5\,\mathrm{pA\,\mu m^{-1}}$ for B and D. (From Korogod *et al.*, 2002.)

density reaches zero in every dendrite, making a large part of the dendritic field a functionally silent zone. Comparison of the downstate and upstate reveals a much more heterogeneous contribution of each individual dendrite to the total somatopetal current in the downstate.

To explore the contribution of each dendritic compartment to the current reaching the soma, we compute the current transfer effectiveness for the downstate and upstate of the electrical bistability of the same motoneuron.

12.5.2 Maps of current transfer effectiveness

The results of the computation are mapped on the 3D image and dendrogram of the arborization (Figure 12.6). In the downstate, the spatial maps of the current transfer effectiveness (Figure 12.6, A and C) reveal that the difference between the most effective proximal parts and the low effectiveness distal regions of the dendritic field is extremely small, from 0 to 0.15 pA μm^{-1}. However, in this narrow dynamic range, the transfer effectiveness varies greatly between different dendritic sites, giving a patchy image of the dendritic field with the most effective patches in the proximal dendritic branches and the least effective ones distributed in the distal dendritic parts. In the upstate, a small peri-somatic zone restricted to only four dendritic stems displays a high transfer effectiveness of −8.5 pA μm^{-1} (Figure 12.6, D) which decreases rapidly to low values with a location-dependent variability. Beyond 100–200 μm from the soma, the whole dendritic field displays zero efficiency and is electrically disconnected from the soma. These spatial patterns (Figure 12.6, B and D) are similar to those of the current density maps illustrated in Figure 12.5, B and D.

Hence, the material of this chapter has shown the 3D location of the electrical domains in the dendritic field and show that they are dependent on changes in the passive membrane resistivity R_m (conductivity $G_m = 1/R_m$) as well as on voltage-dependent membrane properties. We have demonstrated that the dynamic spatial variations of the 3D domains are related to the *metrical asymmetry* of the arborization and to the orientation of metrically asymmetrical parts in 3D space. We have revealed some geometry-related 3D patterns in the electrical structure of the arborization that are related to specific types of neurons. Finally, we have shown features of the 3D electrical structures of the arborizations that can be common to different types of neurons.

References

Bras, H., Gogan, P. and Tyč-Dumont, S. (1987). The dendrites of single brain-stem motoneurons intracellularly labelled with horseradish peroxidase in the cat. Morphological and electrical differences. *Neuroscience*, **22**:947–970.

Bras, H., Korogod, S., Driencourt, Y., Gogan, P. and Tyč-Dumont, S. (1993). Stochastic geometry and electrotonic architecture of dendritic arborization of a brain-stem motoneuron. *Eur. J. Neurosci.*, **5**:1405–1493.

Korogod, S. M., Bras, H., Sarana, V. N., Gogan, P. and Tyč-Dumont, S. (1994). Electrotonic clusters in the dendritic arborisation of abducens motoneurons in the rat. *Eur. J. Neurosci.*, **6**:1517–1527.

Korogod, S. M., Kulagina, I. B., Horcholle-Bossavit, G., Gogan, P. and Tyč-Dumont, S. (2000). Activity-dependent reconfiguration of the effective dendritic field of motoneurons. *J. Comp. Neurol.*, **422**:18–34.

Korogod, S. M., Kulagina, I. B., Kukushka, V. I., Gogan, P. and Tyč-Dumont, S. (2002). Spatial reconfiguration of charge transfer effectiveness in active bistable dendritic arborizations. *Eur. J. Neurosci.*, **16**:2260–2270.

Kulagina, I. B., Korogod, S. M., Horcholle-Bossavit, G., Batini, C. and Tyč-Dumont, S. (2007). The electro-dynamics of the dendritic space in Purkinje cells of the cerebellum. *Arch. Ital. Biol.*, **145**:211–233.

13

Dendritic space as a coder of the temporal output patterns

The dendritic job to process synaptic inputs ends by generating patterns of output discharges. If the site of initiation of action potentials has long been known, the mechanisms by which the axo-somatic trigger zone is finally put into action is an open question. A 60-year-old large consensus admits the simple explanation: the current shifts the voltage at the initial segment and when a threshold is reached, the neuron fires. The reasons for the numerous different types of output patterns observed from a single neuron are skipped and remain unknown. How the output patterns are formed by the electrical dendritic arborization with non-linear, active membrane is explained in this chapter.

We select two types of neurons with clearly different geometry and cocktails of voltage-dependent channels in their dendrites, and simulate generation of output discharge patterns in response to tonic activation of synaptic inputs distributed over the dendritic membrane to find out the rules that govern the neuronal code.

13.1 Terminology to describe the repertoire of neuronal discharges

We propose the following terminology to describe the types of electrical activity of neurons that we observe in our models.

Elementary electrical event at the neuron output (axon) is a single action potential (spike) or a burst of action potentials. Other examples of elementary events recorded from the soma or dendrites are slow depolarization waves or postsynaptic potentials.

Burst of action potentials is a group of sequential action potentials separated by the same or different time intervals, the duration of which is compatible with the refractoriness period. Examples are groups of two (doublet), three (triplet) or four (quadruplet) action potentials.

Pattern is a certain sequence of elementary electrical events.

Auto-rhythmical pattern is a certain periodically repeating sequence of identical or different elementary electrical events.

Continuous discharge is a pattern formed by long-lasting sequence of action potentials with equal inter-spike intervals.

Repertoire of electrical activity is a set of different patterns which are generated by a neuron in certain conditions (e.g. during tonic synaptic activation with intensities in a certain range).

Although these definitions are not absolutely rigorous, they are sufficient for comparison of different neurons in the richness of their repertoires. If the time intervals between elementary events change insignificantly so that it is possible to consider the activity type unchanged (e.g. repeating quadruplets or repeating triplets), then it is taken as a variation of activity of the same type. A new pattern is thought to occur if, for instance, a sequence of triplets changes to a sequence of doublets or to a repeating sequence of combined 'doublet-triplets'. The repertoire is considered to be more rich if a neuron is able to generate a greater number of different patterns with changes of synaptic activation in the same range of intensities.

13.2 Geometry-induced features of Purkinje cell discharges

Two types of models of the Purkinje neuron with active dendrites are considered. The first type has a soma, axon and dendrites active, due to the presence of corresponding sets of voltage-dependent channels. In the second type, the soma and axon are passive, to mimic the blockade of the trigger zone, and the dendrites remain active, although with a shorter list of channel types.

13.2.1 Model with active dendrites, soma and axon

The types and distribution of the voltage-dependent channels are the same as in earlier models described by Miyasho *et al.* (2001) and De Schutter and Bower (1994), in which the equations and parameters describing these channels, as well as the relevant references can be found. The model contains channels conducting the following 13 currents: fast inactivating sodium (NaF), persistent sodium (NaP), P-type calcium (CaP2), T-type calcium (CaT), E-type calcium (CaE), anomalous rectification potassium (Kh), delayed rectification (Hodgkin–Huxley type) potassium (Khh), persistent M-type potassium (KM), A-type potassium (KA), D-type potassium (KD), BK-type calcium-dependent potassium (KC3), K-type calcium-dependent potassium (K23) and the passive leak current (Leak). The channels of CaP2, CaT, CaE, Khh, KM, KA, KD, KC3, K23 and Leak currents are present in the dendritic membrane. The somatic membrane contains the channels of NaF,

NaP, CaP2, CaT, CaE, Khh, KM, KA, Kh and Leak currents. The axon hillock and initial segment contain the passive leak and voltage-dependent channels (Hodgkin–Huxley type): fast inactivating sodium and non-inactivating potassium channels. The Ranvier nodes of the myelinated stem axon contain Hodgkin–Huxley type fast sodium channels at high density and the passive leak. The myelinated segments are passive. The somato-dendritic part of the model neuron also contains a mechanism of intracellular calcium dynamics, which takes into account calcium entry into the cytoplasm through plasmolemmal channels and extrusion from the submembrane cytosol layer (e.g. by action of the pumps and by diffusion to the bulk of the intracellular space) with a certain time constant.

In all computation experiments, a homogeneously distributed tonic activation of the dendritic synaptic inputs is simulated by introducing voltage-independent (AMPA-type glutamatergic) spatially homogeneous synaptic conductivity G_s associated with the reversal potential $E_s = 0\,\mathrm{mV}$. Certain constant values of G_s correspond to different intensities of the tonic synaptic activation. The cytoplasm resistivity is $R_i = 250\ \Omega \cdot \mathrm{cm}$. The membrane specific capacitance C_m is $0.8\ \mu\mathrm{F\,cm}^{-2}$ in the smooth dendrites and $1.5\ \mu\mathrm{F\,cm}^{-2}$ in the spiny dendrites (see Miyasho *et al.*, 2001 and Kulagina *et al.*, 2007 for details).

13.2.2 Output discharge repertoire and dendritic states

In the models of the Purkinje neuron with the 'complete' set of voltage-gated and calcium-dependent channels, including all fast discharge mechanisms, the repertoire of electrical activity and the role of dendritic geometry in the formation of electrical patterns are analyzed with the following stimulation protocol. The temporal and spatial patterns of electrical activity are studied at different intensities of tonic activation of excitatory AMPA-type synaptic conductivity, expressed in $\mu\mathrm{S\,cm}^{-2}$ homogeneously distributed over the dendrites.

At synaptic intensities subthreshold for action potentials, a membrane depolarization is generated in the dendrites. This depolarization is spatially heterogeneous and is greatest in the most distal dendritic sites, decaying towards the soma with unequal rates along asymmetrical dendritic paths. Since there is no propagating discharge, this activity does not count as an *output* pattern.

A typical repertoire of auto-rhythmical electrical activity of Purkinje neurons is illustrated by Figures 13.1 and 13.2 for the example of cell P1. For this cell, the threshold of action potentials is reached at a synaptic intensity of $47\ \mu\mathrm{S\,cm}^{-2}$. At synaptic conductivity (activation intensity) values ranging between 47 and $65\ \mu\mathrm{S\,cm}^{-2}$, the modelled neuron generates a sequence of repeating quadruplets (illustrated at $50\ \mu\mathrm{S\,cm}^{-2}$ in Figure 13.1). The output activity is a sequential repetition of the same burst which includes four action potentials with shorter intervals

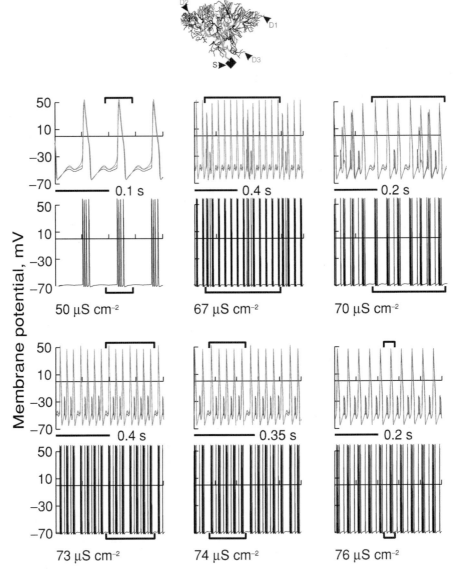

Figure 13.1 (Plate 9) Repertoire of electrical activity generated in the dendrites (upper curves) and axon (lower curves in black) of the cerebellar Purkinje neurons (P1) with active conductances at different intensities of tonic activation of the excitatory synaptic inputs homogeneously distributed over the dendritic arborization. Calibration bars: time, s. Ordinates: membrane potential, mV. The tonic synaptic activation of the dendrites is simulated by introducing a homogeneous synaptic conductivity (given in $\mu S\ cm^{-2}$ near corresponding plots). Horizontal brackets above and below recordings envelop the repeating sequence of the elementary electrical events which correspond to the action potentials and their bursts. The reversal potential of the synaptic current equals 0 mV. Red, green and blue curves: recordings of the membrane potential from sites D1, D2 and D3 shown on the 3D representation of the Purkinje neuron (top). The sites are selected in the sectors of the low, medium and high relative effectiveness of the somatopetal current transfer (L, M and H in Figure 12.1, P1). (From I. Kulagina, Dnipropetrovsk National University.)

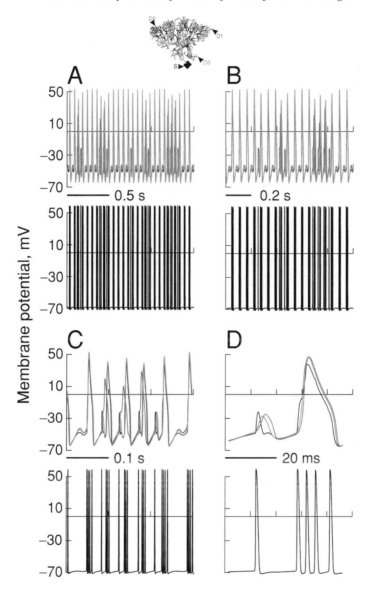

Figure 13.2 (Plate 10) Same as Figure 13.1 but during generation of a pseudo-stochastic pattern at a synaptic intensity of 68 μS cm^{-2}. Fragments of the recording are shown at different timescales (A, B, C, D) to facilitate the comparison of the events in different parts of the cell. (From I. Kulagina, Dnipropetrovsk National University.)

between the first, second and third spikes and longer intervals between the third and fourth spikes. In the given range, the greater the synaptic intensity, the shorter the inter-spike and inter-burst intervals are (greater frequency of bursts and spikes in a burst). This is an example of the same activity pattern but with variation of the parameters of the activity.

Further increase of synaptic intensity in a narrow range of 66 to 67 μS cm^{-2} leads to a dramatic increase in the pattern complexity: there is an increase both in the number of different elementary events in the repeating sequence and in the duration of the sequence. For instance, at the intensity of 67 μS cm^{-2}, the repeating sequence includes as many as 13 elementary events: a quadruplet (event 1); a spike-quadruplet complex (event 2); five quadruplets in series (events 3 to 7); a spike-triplet complex (event 8); a spike-quadruplet complex (event 9) and four quadruplets in series (events 10 to 13). The duration of this repeating 13-event sequence (and, correspondingly, the repetition period) is about 700 ms. At 68 μS cm^{-2}, it is difficult to determine the repeating sequence because of the significant variability in sequential elementary events (Figure 13.2), so that, in this case, the activity is classified as quasi-stochastic (may be an example of the deterministic chaos). The repetition is not noticed even after a 12 second observation.

With the synaptic intensity increased above 68 μS cm^{-2}, one can again observe certain repeating sequences of the elementary events which form more or less complex compositions. For instance, at 69 μS cm^{-2}, the repeating sequence is composed of three bursts: two quadruplets and one spike-quadruplet complex (not shown). At 70 μS cm^{-2}, the repeating sequence includes seven bursts: 1 and 2 are quadruplets; 3 is a spike-quadruplet complex; 4 is a quadruplet; 5 and 6 are two spike-triplet complexes with slightly different inter-spike intervals and finally 7 is a spike-quadruplet complex (Figure 13.1). At 73 μS cm^{-2}, the repeating sequence also includes seven elementary events: initially it is a quadruplet (event 1) which is followed by two spike-quadruplet complexes (events 2 and 3), then, with a longer interval (about 50 ms), there is again a quadruplet (event 4) followed by three more spike-quadruplet complexes (events 5 to 7). At 74 μS cm^{-2}, the repeating sequence also includes five elementary events: 1 is a quadruplet and 2–4 are three spike-quadruplet complexes (the duration, i.e. the repetition period of the sequence, is about 250 ms). At 76 μS cm^{-2}, the sequence is significantly simplified down to a spike-quadruplet complex. Further increase in the synaptic intensity over a wide range of values is accompanied with a further simplification of the repeating sequence to being composed of only one elementary event. At values of 85 to 700 μS cm^{-2}, this repeating sequence is a spike-triplet complex. At 2 mS cm^{-2} it is a spike-doublet complex. At 5 mS cm^{-2}, continuous firing is observed with the period modulated by sinusoidal oscillations of the membrane potential in the dendrites.

At $7\,\mathrm{mS\,cm^{-2}}$, such a continuous firing activity has a constant period (inter-spike interval) and at that time a persistent high-level depolarization is observed in the dendrites.

We conclude that, in the cerebellar Purkinje neurons, it is possible to determine three ranges of intensity of the distributed tonic synaptic activation for which the output activity patterns of different complexity are observed:

(1) The low range (or the state of low membrane conductivity), which is characterized by a relatively simple pattern formed by a low-frequency periodical repetition of only one certain elementary event. In the case of cell P1, it is the range from 47 to 65 $\mu\mathrm{S\,cm^{-2}}$ and the repeating event is a quadruplet of spikes with a greater repetition frequency corresponding to greater synaptic intensity.
(2) The medium range (or the state of intermediate membrane conductivity), for which characteristics are complex patterns formed by periodical repetition of multiple elementary events of diverse composition. In the example of cell P1, it is the range from 66 to 80 $\mu\mathrm{S\,cm^{-2}}$. With increasing intensity in this range, the number of repeating events in a sequence first increases from 2 to 13 and then decreases to 2. The types of the elementary events which appear in the repeating sequences are also more diverse. They are quadruplets and triplets as well as 'spike-quadruplet' and 'spike-triplet' complexes.
(3) The high range (or the state of high membrane conductivity), for which the characteristic patterns are also simple, formed by a single-type one-event repeating sequence, but following with a much higher frequency in contrast to the low range. In the example of Purkinje cell P1, this range corresponds to synaptic conductivity values greater than $80\,\mu\mathrm{S\,cm^{-2}}$ and the unique repeating elementary event is either spike-triplet complex (in subrange from about 80 to 700 $\mu\mathrm{S\,cm^{-2}}$), spike-doublet, simple doublet or finally a spike, i.e. continuous firing (in the higher subrange).

13.2.3 Dendritic events during output discharges

A critical observation is the electrical states of active dendrites in the regions which are characterized as having low, medium and high effectiveness of the somatopetal current transfer in the passive configuration (red, green and blue recordings at sites D1, D2 and D3, in Figures 13.1 and 13.2).

When regular simple periodical patterns are generated at low (50 $\mu\mathrm{S\,cm^{-2}}$) or high (76 $\mu\mathrm{S\,cm^{-2}}$) synaptic intensities, then the membrane potential transitions between downstate and upstate are simultaneous at these different sites and the levels of the upstate and downstate voltage remain equal from cycle to cycle. Closely overlapping traces indicate that the different domains of the arborization have very similar voltages at each phase of the activity, i.e. they are in very similar electrical states with a smaller difference in the upstate and a greater difference in the downstate. In other words, during generation of simple regular patterns, the membrane voltage changes over the whole dendritic arborization almost homogeneously. A small electrical heterogeneity in the dendritic space is due to a certain, relatively small phase shift between periodical events at different sites.

The *spatial dendritic signature* of complex patterns observed at medium-range synaptic intensities is essentially different. For instance, consider a complex pattern of seven repeating events obtained at an intensity of $70\,\mu S\,cm^{-2}$ (Figure 13.1). The difference between red, green and blue traces is very big, especially during the generation of the last three events in the sequence. Another noteworthy detail of the pattern is the significant variation of the upstate depolarization levels from one event to another in the sequence, observed at each recording site, but especially big at the low-effectiveness site D1 (red trace). Similar features are clearly seen in the most complex pattern at $68\,\mu S\,cm^{-2}$ (Figure 13.2, C). Hence, during generation of complex patterns, there is an essential heterogeneity of electrical states over the whole arborization with a noticeable difference between parts which are also most different in their passive transfer properties.

It is worthwhile to remember that the metrical asymmetry was shown to be the main reason for the difference in the passive transfer over dendrites with homogeneous membrane properties. Based on these observations, we assume that the metrical asymmetry is a common reason for the difference between asymmetrical parts of the dendritic arborization in both passive transfer properties and dynamic regenerative activity. This suggestion is favoured by the fact that the difference in both respects is small at low and high intensities of synaptic activation (i.e. in the low- and high-conductance states, respectively) and is big at synaptic intensities in the intermediate range (i.e. in the mid-conductance state). To summarize, equalization of electrical state in dendritic space is associated with a better synchronization of activity of different parts of the arborization over time.

13.2.4 Model with active dendrites but passive soma and axon

Here, the model is modified. The soma and axon are made purely passive (the membrane conductivity $G_m = 677.25\,\mu S\,cm^{-2}$ associated with resting potential $E_p = -65\,mV$) and the set of dendritic channels is reduced to five: CaP2, Khh, KA, KC3 and Leak. The excluded dendritic channels are those conducting small currents, which add minor details to the main oscillatory activity. All other channels, calcium dynamics and AMPA-type synaptic conductivity distributed over the dendrites are kept the same.

The data described above indicate that the generation of auto-rhythmical patterns of different complexities is related to certain structure-dependent changes in electrical states of different parts of the dendritic arborization, which can be considered as the *spatial dendritic signature* of certain electrical events occurring at the cell output. However, there can be alternatives in defining the neuron parts in which the main pattern is formed. One possible scenario is that the temporal pattern is initiated in the axo-somatic trigger zone and then propagates along the axon and back-invades the dendrites. This back invasion spreads differently along different, particularly asymmetrical dendritic paths as was earlier observed in the model of a reconstructed abducens motoneuron (Korogod *et al.*, 1996). According to an alternative scenario, the dendritic arborization itself plays the pattern-forming role: different dendritic parts change their states of low and high depolarization and supply the trigger zone with different somatopetal currents, which are transformed into corresponding sequences of action potentials.

In the following series of computer experiments, the hypothesis of the principal pattern-forming role of the dendrites is tested. The whole axo-somatic membrane of the Purkinje neuron is made passive by switching off the fast discharge mechanisms. In other words, the voltage-dependent channels in the soma and axon are blocked, but those in the dendrites remain in operation, together with the mechanisms of intracellular calcium dynamics. In these conditions, the trigger zone is actually absent and any auto-rhythmical pattern has exclusively a dendritic origin. The results obtained in these conditions are shown in Figures 13.3 to 13.6.

As in the previous simulations (Figures 13.1 and 13.2), the same tonic activation of AMPA-type synaptic conductivity homogeneously distributed over the dendrites causes oscillatory depolarization potentials in the modified Purkinje neuron model. The shape and frequency of the oscillations depend on synaptic intensity (Figure 13.3).

At low supra-threshold intensity of the tonic activation (synaptic conductivity of $50\,\mu S\,cm^{-2}$ for neuron P1), the dendrites generate periodical relatively low-amplitude depolarization waves from -60 to -30 mV and a period of about 40–50 ms which are conducted passively into the soma and decay almost to the resting potential along the axon (Figure 13.3). At a greater intensity of activation ($54\,\mu S\,cm^{-2}$), the periodical pattern changes: the dendrites generate a relatively low-frequency (period about 90 ms) repeating sequence composed of a low-amplitude (extent from -40 to -25 mV) faster wave followed by a high-amplitude (extent from -75 to $+60$ mV) slower wave of depolarization. With a further increased intensity of $58\,\mu S\,cm^{-2}$, there are two low-amplitude and one high-amplitude waves in the repeating sequence. The spatial picture of the activity recorded in the same three sites located in the regions of low, medium and high relative transfer effectiveness (red, green and blue lines in the upper records of Figures 13.3 and 13.5) indicates that the membrane potentials oscillate with the same frequency, but with a certain phase shift. Each depolarization wave is generated first at the site of low electrical effectiveness (red line, then at the site

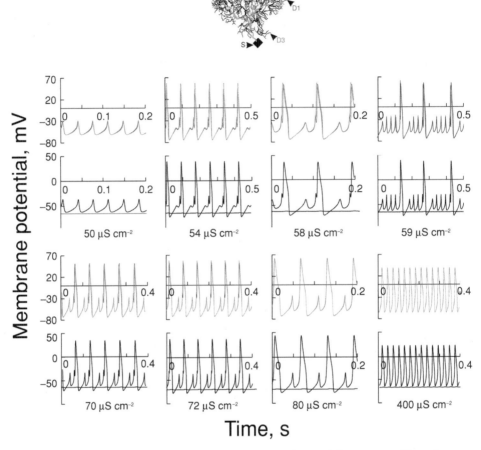

Figure 13.3 (Plate 11) Repertoire of the slow electrical activity generated in active dendrites (upper coloured curves) and passive soma and axon (lower black curves) of the cerebellar Purkinje neuron P1 (top) at different intensities (given in $\mu S\ cm^{-2}$) of tonic activation of the excitatory synaptic inputs homogeneously distributed over the dendritic arborization. Abscissas: time, s. Ordinates: the membrane potential, mV. The colours of the recordings of the dendritic potentials correspond to those in Figures 13.1 and 13.2. (From I. Kulagina, Dnipropetrovsk National University.)

of intermediate effectiveness (green line), then at the high-effectiveness site (blue line) and finally at the soma (the black lower records of Figures 13.3 and 13.5). At different sites, the amplitudes of the waves differ from each other, but at each site the amplitudes are constant in time. With the activation intensity increased to $59\ \mu S\ cm^{-2}$, the pattern is complicated further and its spatial picture changes significantly (Figure 13.3). The pattern observed in these conditions can be qualified as quasi-stochastic, because it is not possible to detect a certain repeating sequence of waves even during an observation as long as 12 seconds (Figure 13.4).

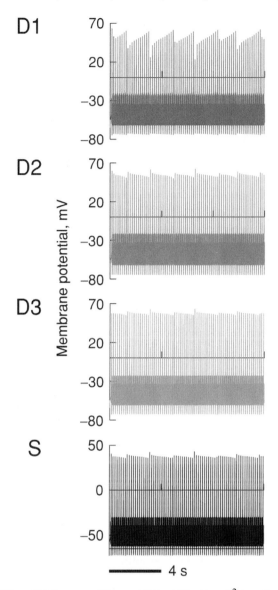

Figure 13.4 (Plate 12) Same as Figure 13.3 at $59\,\mu\mathrm{S\,cm^{-2}}$ but the recordings at sites D1–D3 and S are shown separately (see Figure 13.1 legend for labelling) and during longer time. The repeating sequence is not detected even during an observation time as long as 12 s, which may mean a pseudo-stochastic pattern of slow oscillations of the membrane potential. Time calibration bar: s. Ordinates: membrane potential, mV. (From I. Kulagina, Dnipropetrovsk National University.)

In this case, the spatial dendritic picture of electrical activity (Figure 13.3) is:

(1) An irregular oscillatory process is observed which is a combination of higher-frequency, low-amplitude and lower-frequency, high-amplitude waves of depolarization in all derivations.
(2) The low-amplitude oscillations have a more regular periodicity. The high-amplitude oscillations have a noticeably irregular period which is not related to the period of the low-amplitude waves: during the time interval between two consecutive high-amplitude waves, three or four low-amplitude waves are generated.
(3) Depending on phase relationship between the low- and high-frequency oscillations, the amplitude of the low-frequency wave is augmented if it occurs on the rising phase of the high-frequency depolarization, or is noticeably reduced if it is generated during the falling phase of the high-frequency wave. As a consequence, the amplitude of the low-frequency oscillations vary significantly.

Especially noticeable variations are observed at the site belonging to the dendritic region of low relative effectiveness of the somatopetal current transfer (D1). At the sites situated on the subtrees with medium (D2) or high (D3) current transfer effectiveness and at the soma (S), the low-frequency waves have smaller variations of amplitude, but the period of these waves varies noticeably.

Further increase in intensity of the synaptic activation to 70 or 72 μS cm^{-2} leads again to a regular rhythm and constant amplitudes of both high-frequency and low-frequency oscillations. At 70 μS cm^{-2}, the phase shift between the oscillations in differently effective parts of the arborization is conspicuous. In this case, the repeating sequence includes two low-amplitude waves and one high-amplitude wave. At 72 μS cm^{-2}, the phase shift becomes smaller and the difference between the second low-amplitude wave and the high-amplitude wave is reduced. At 80 μS cm^{-2}, these differences are almost undetectable and the repeating sequence is a composition of two waves: one low-amplitude and one high-amplitude wave. With increase of intensity (e.g. up to 400 μS cm^{-2}, Figure 13.3), the low-amplitude waves disappear, the frequency of the high-amplitude depolarization waves increases and their amplitudes decrease. With further increased intensity of the tonic synaptic excitation, the depolarization waves approach sinusoidal oscillations and their amplitude decreases significantly. The membrane potential oscillates almost sinusoidally about the level, which is significantly shifted to high depolarization. Finally, a high-intensity activation leads to development of steady spatially heterogeneous depolarization without any oscillations (not shown).

Comparison of this slow auto-rhythmical activity with the oscillatory bursting discharges observed when the fast discharge mechanisms are not blocked shows that, over time, the faster low-amplitude wave of depolarization corresponds

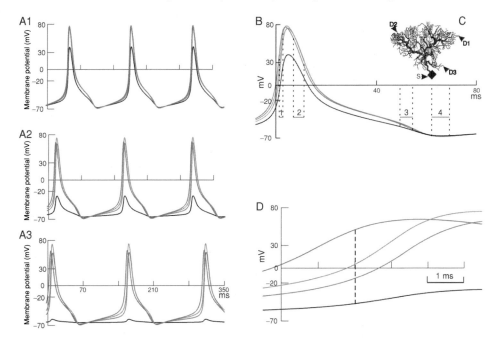

Figure 13.5 (Plate 13) Oscillatory potentials generated by the Purkinje cell (C) with active dendrites receiving distributed tonic synaptic excitation. A1: Regular auto-oscillations computed with axo-somatic passive membrane resistivity $G_m = 677.25\,\mu S\,cm^{-2}$ and recorded from the soma (black trace) and three dendritic sites (red, green and blue traces). B: A single expanded oscillatory cycle extracted from A1 to show the phase-shift of voltages at the soma S (in black) and at three dendritic sites D1 (in red), D2 (in green) and D3 (in blue) localized as indicated by arrowheads in C. The four horizontal segments labelled 1–4 and the vertical dotted lines indicate the phases of the oscillatory potential during which snapshots were collected and depicted in Figure 13.6. A2 and A3: Same recordings as in A1 but computed with $G_m = 6.7725$ and $67.725\,mS\,cm^{-2}$, respectively, to show the differences in amplitudes and shift in time as compared to A1. D: A single oscillatory cycle extracted from A2 with an expanded timescale to show better the differences in phase and amplitude (dotted lines) between the recordings. Abscissae: time, ms. Note the different timescales. Ordinates: the membrane potential, mV. (From Kulagina *et al.*, 2007.)

approximately to the single action potential and the following high-amplitude slow wave corresponds to a burst with a smaller or greater number of action potentials.

13.2.5 Spatial dendritic signature of the oscillatory temporal pattern

Figure 13.5 shows oscillations of the membrane potentials recorded from the soma and three different dendritic sites (labelled S, D1, D2 and D3 on the 3D image of the arborization in insert C) of the Purkinje model with passive soma and axon. The computations are performed for three different values of passive membrane conductivity G_m of the axo-somatic region providing a passive leak for the active dendrites to prove the robustness of the dendritic oscillatory pattern.

In A1, a fragment of activity at $G_m = 677.25 \, \mu\text{S cm}^{-2}$ is shown. The four recordings are of different amplitudes, of slightly different shapes and occur with a shift in time relative to each other. A single oscillation extracted from A1 is shown in B in an expanded timescale to better illustrate the shift. The depolarization potential at D1 (red trace) develops first, having a peak amplitude of 76.6 mV. The second potential is recorded from D2 (green trace) with the highest amplitude of 79.0 mV and is followed by the potential from D3 (blue trace) of 75 mV in amplitude. The delayed potential recorded from the soma (black trace) has a peak amplitude of 40 mV. In A2 ($G_m = 6.7725 \, \text{mS cm}^{-2}$), the dendritic recordings are similar to those in A1, but with a slightly larger shift in time while the somatic recording displays a much smaller amplitude, reaching -40 mV. The current delivered from the dendrites to the soma with a lower resistance produces a smaller voltage drop. The difference in time and amplitude between the four recorded potentials (extracted from one oscillation in A2) is best illustrated in D, with an expanded timescale at the start of the rising phase of the oscillation. The main result is that the recording D1 preceded D2 and D3 by several milliseconds. The difference in amplitudes between the potentials recorded at the given sites S, D1, D2 and D3 of the dendritic arborization and at a given moment in time (dashed lines) of the oscillation are, for example, as large as about 100 mV between D1 and soma S. In A3 ($G_m = 67.725 \, \text{mS cm}^{-2}$), a larger difference in amplitude between dendritic and somatic recordings occurs. There is also a difference in amplitude and a larger shift in time with respect to the values observed in A1 and A2. The demonstration that the oscillatory potentials are ordered in time is an important finding that facilitates further understanding of the dynamics of the membrane potentials in the dendritic field observed in space.

Figure 13.6 shows successive snapshots of the map of the membrane potentials over the dendritic arborization taken during the four phases of the oscillatory cycle indicated by labels 1, 2, 3 and 4 in Figure 13.5, B. The sequence, in which the dendritic domains change their consecutive colours, allows identification of the sequence of changes in the membrane potential and derivation of the phase relationships of the events at these domains. This proper procedure allows the demonstration of the split of the dendritic arborization into domains of different voltage transients. Noteworthy, these domains correspond to those identified in the passive configuration in the steady state (Figure 12.1, P1).

During the first phase of the cycle starting at the beginning of the rising phase of the potential ($t = 1.2 \, \text{ms}$), almost the entire dendritic arborization is set at a

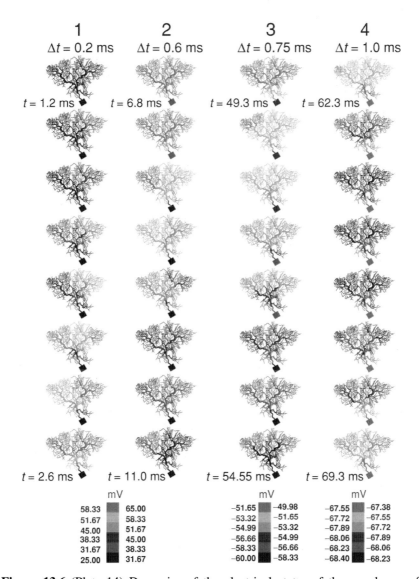

Figure 13.6 (Plate 14) Dynamics of the electrical states of the membrane of the Purkinje cell arborization. Snapshots of the dendritic maps of the membrane potentials taken during phases 1 to 4 of the oscillatory cycle shown under the potential in Figure 13.5, B. Columns 1 to 4 show eight snapshots taken with equal time step Δt from top to bottom. Column 1 corresponds to the rising phase of the potential, starting at $t = 1.2$ ms and ending at $t = 2.6$ ms, snapshots taken every 0.2 ms. Column 2 corresponds to the falling phase of the plateau potential, starting at $t = 6.8$ ms and ending at $t = 11.0$ ms, snapshots taken every 0.6 ms. Columns 3 and 4 correspond to increasing ($\Delta t = 0.75$ ms) and decreasing ($\Delta t = 1.0$ ms) inter-plateau hyperpolarizations, starting at $t = 49.3$ ms and 62.3 ms and ending at $t = 54.55$ ms and $t = 69.3$ ms, respectively. Membrane potential in mV is colour-coded by the same six-colour palette in different ranges: from 25 to 65 mV for columns 1 and 2, from -49.98 to 60 mV for column 3 and from -67.38 to -68.4 mV for column 4. (From Kulagina *et al.*, 2007.) Interactive detailed considerations of the animation are provided by NeuronViewer tool with data file PurkinjeP1.dat available at URL www.cambridge.org/9780521896771.

potential between 25.0 to 31.67 mV except a tiny north-east domain between 31.67 to 38.33 mV (Figure 13.6, column 1). The following snapshots in the column show that the shift to higher values involves first the north-east domain (38.33 mV). Then, the arborization is split into successive dendritic domains with low to high voltages which are ordered in space. The voltage reaches the highest values (58.33 to 65 mV) first in the north-east domain (the sixth snapshot in column 1). A state of fully depolarized dendritic arborization (Figure 13.6, column 2) is reached just before the beginning of phase 2 (indicated in Figure 13.5, B), corresponding to the start of the repolarizing phase of the potential ($t = 6.8$ ms). At that given moment, the soma is depolarized between 31.67 and 38.33 mV. On the way back to repolarization (column 2), the split between domains occurs again in an inverse order to reach voltages between 38.33 and 25 mV (the end of column 2). At the beginning of phase 3 (Figure 13.6, column 3, $t = 49.3$ ms), the arborization is hyperpolarized between -49.98 and -51.65 mV, except some small domains near the soma. During phase 3, the arborization is again divided into domains showing potentials between -51.65 and -60 mV with regional differences of some tenths of mV. During phase 4 (Figure 13.6, column 4, $t = 62.3$ ms), successive dendritic domains are still changing towards hyperpolarization, but the differences between dendritic parts are reduced to only 1 mV (-67.55 to -68.23 mV). Then, a new cycle starts with the same successive spatial patterns of splits (not shown). The turnover of the regional different polarizations of the dendritic membrane lasts the duration of one cycle. One important finding is the fact that the same dendritic sector in the arborization displays a difference in voltage as high as about 130 mV during a single oscillation (see Figure 13.5, D). For example, the north-east domain, which displays 58 to 65 mV at the beginning of the falling phase of the oscillation (row 2), is hyperpolarized to -68 mV at the end of the oscillatory cycle (row 4).

Several features of the spatial maps of the oscillatory depolarization waves are remarkable. The rising phase of the depolarization is steeper than the falling phase (Figure 13.5). During generation of this auto-rhythmical activity, the dendritic arborization behaves as a complex spatial oscillator with synchronous but not in-phase changes in the membrane potential in different subtrees (Figures 13.5 and 13.6). In different parts of the dendritic arborization, the oscillations take place with the same frequency (synchrony), but are phase-shifted in a certain structure-dependent order. During each oscillatory cycle, the depolarization increases first in the dendritic sectors that are characterized by a low relative passive transfer effectiveness and then, the depolarization wave develops sequentially in the sectors with intermediate and high transfer effectiveness. The decay of the depolarization occurs in the same sequence, from low- to high-effectiveness sectors. As the ranking of the dendritic sectors according to their transfer effectiveness is clearly correlated with the metrical asymmetry of the corresponding subtrees, there are reasons to reckon that the same geometrical factors also determine the phase relationships between oscillations of the membrane potential in different sectors and thus the formation of the entire spatial-temporal pattern of the electrical activity of the Purkinje model.

13.3 Geometry-dependent repertoire of pyramidal cell activity

The types and distribution of the membrane conductivities in our simulations of discharge patterns of neocortical pyramidal neurons are the same as in earlier models of this cell type (Mainen and Sejnowski, 1996, and references therein). In short, the dendritic membrane contains the channels conducting the following currents: fast inactivating sodium (Hamill *et al.*, 1991; Mainen *et al.*, 1995), high-voltage activated (HVA) inactivating calcium (Reuveni *et al.*, 1993), muscarinic (M-type) potassium (Gutfreund *et al.*, 1995), calcium-dependent potassium (Reuveni *et al.*, 1993) and the passive leak current. The soma, axon hillock and initial segment contain the same channel types as the dendrites and, in addition, the delayed rectification non-inactivating potassium channels of Hodgkin–Huxley type (Hamill *et al.*, 1991; Mainen *et al.*, 1995). In the axon, the myelinated segments contain passive leak conductivity of a very low value and the Ranvier nodes contain fast inactivating sodium conductivity (Hamill *et al.*, 1991; Mainen *et al.*, 1995) of a high value and passive leak conductivity. The cytoplasm resistivity $R_i = 150\,\Omega \cdot \text{cm}$ is homogeneous over the whole cell. The membrane capacitance is $C_m = 0.75\,\mu\text{F}\,\text{cm}^{-2}$ everywhere except at myelinated segments of the axon $(C_m = 0.04\,\mu\text{F}\,\text{cm}^{-2})$. The somato-dendritic part of the model contains a calcium dynamics mechanism similar to that mentioned above in the description of the Purkinje cell model. The equations and parameters describing the membrane currents and intracellular calcium dynamics are taken from Mainen and Sejnowski (1996) with the corrections given by the authors in the model database ModelDB at URL: http://senselab.med.yale.edu/senselab/modeldb/ShowModel.asp?model=2488.

13.3.1 Arborization size and electrical repertoire

The repertoire of activity of the simulated pyramidal neurons is studied using tonic excitatory synaptic activation homogeneously distributed over dendrites with active conductances. Such activation is simulated by introducing spatially homogeneous voltage-independent synaptic conductance (analogous to AMPA-type glutamatergic conductance). The spatial-temporal picture of electrical activity of the neuron is recorded at different intensities of activation.

The main result of this series of computation experiments is the observation of the dependence of the electrical patterns on the dendritic asymmetry and the changes in the repertoire with changing the synaptic conductance states. As for the Purkinje neuron (Figure 13.1), three ranges of homogeneous synaptic activation are defined that are associated with discharge patterns of different complexity. They are low, medium and high ranges of synaptic conductivity. Simple patterns composed of one repeating elementary event are characteristic of the low and high ranges, whereas at the medium range intensity the neuron generates several complex patterns composed of two or much more elementary events, which are often of different types. It is noteworthy that the limits of these three ranges in the pyramidal neurons are significantly (several times or even one order) lower compared to those determined by the pattern complexity changes in the Purkinje neurons.

A typical example is illustrated by Figure 13.7, which shows the recordings from the axon of the reconstructed pyramidal neuron C1 taken from the work of Mainen and Sejnowski (1996).

For generation of the auto-rhythmical activity, the threshold value is $4.5 \, \mu S \, cm^{-2}$. The modelled pyramidal neuron generates a rather simple pattern that is the repetition of a triplet of spikes with an approximately 1 s interval. When the synaptic intensity exceeds $9 \, \mu S \, cm^{-2}$, the pattern becomes more complex in terms of both the number and diversity of events in the repeating sequence. At a synaptic conductivity of $9 \, \mu S \, cm^{-2}$, two elementary events repeat: a triplet followed by a doublet. At $10 \, \mu S \, cm^{-2}$, the repeating sequence includes five elementary events: events 1 to 4 are four doublets with somewhat different inter-spike intervals and event 5 is a triplet. At $11 \, \mu S \, cm^{-2}$, a sequence of another five events repeats: two individual spikes (events 1 and 2) followed by three doublets (events 3 to 5). At $12 \, \mu S \, cm^{-2}$, the repeating sequence numbers seven events: a doublet (event 1), four individual spikes (events 2 to 5), again a doublet (event 6) and finally a triplet (event 7). At $13 \, \mu S \, cm^{-2}$, it is practically impossible to determine a repeating sequence because of the diversity of sequential combinations of elementary events which include individual spikes, doublets and sometimes triplets. Such a pattern is considered to be quasi-stochastic. Further increase in the synaptic intensity leads to regularization and simplification of the pattern, which is a high-frequency repetition of a doublet at $15 \, \mu S \, cm^{-2}$ and becomes a continuous discharge of action potentials with a constant inter-spike interval at $20 \, \mu S \, cm^{-2}$ and more.

13.3.2 Spatial dendritic signatures of the temporal output patterns

The formation of spatial and temporal electrical patterns in the dendrites can be comprehended by comparing the recordings made from different parts of the arborization (A) during generation of aperiodical (B) and high-frequency periodical discharges (C) in Figure 13.8. The activity is recorded at the soma, at two

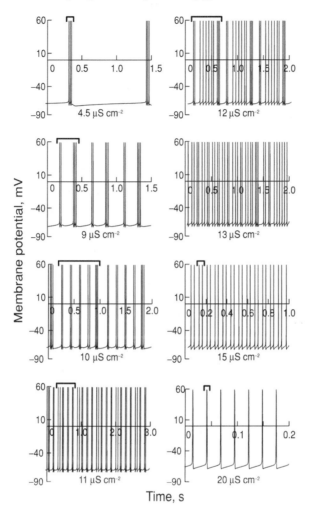

Figure 13.7 Repertoire of electrical activity generated at the output of the pyramidal neuron C1 with active dendrites at different intensities of tonic activation of the excitatory synaptic inputs, homogeneously distributed over the dendritic arborization. Abscissae: time, s. Ordinates: the membrane potential in mV at the distal segment of the axon. Each horizontal bracket envelops the repeating sequence of the elementary electrical events (action potentials and/or their bursts). The tonic synaptic activation of the dendrites is simulated by introducing a homogeneous synaptic conductivity (given in $\mu S\,cm^{-2}$ below each plot). The reversal potential of the synaptic current equals 0 mV. (From I. Kulagina, Dnipropetrovsk National University.)

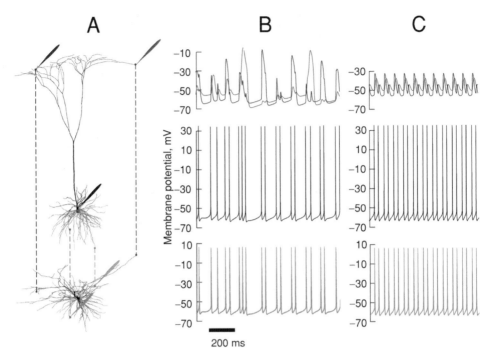

Figure 13.8 (Plate 15) An example of simultaneous recording of electrical activity in different parts of the pyramidal neuron C1. A: Location of the recording sites on two projections of the dendritic arborization (side and top views) in the soma (black pointer), asymmetrical apical dendrites (blue and magenta pointers) and basal dendrites (green and yellow pointers). B and C: Recordings of the membrane potential (ordinates: mV) during generation of, respectively, pseudo-stochastic discharge pattern with a synaptic intensity of $13\,\mu S\,cm^{-2}$ and a high-frequency sequence of doublets of action potentials with a synaptic intensity of $15\,\mu S\,cm^{-2}$. The colours of the curves correspond to those of the recording site pointers in A. Time calibration bar: 200 ms. (From I. Kulagina, Dnipropetrovsk National University.) Interactive detailed considerations of the animation are provided by NeuronViewer tool with data files PyramidalB.dat and PyramidalC.dat available at URL www.cambridge.org/9780521896771.

sites in highly asymmetrical apical branches and at two sites in different basal dendrites.

A quasi-stochastic output pattern (B) is generated by cell C1 at synaptic intensities close to $13\,\mu S\,cm^{-2}$. In the soma, it is an aperiodical sequence of such elementary events as individual spikes and their doublets or, rarely, triplets (Figure 13.8, B). A similar pattern is recorded from the basal dendrites, although the spikes have lower amplitudes. Significantly different patterns are simultaneously recorded from the asymmetrical apical dendrites. When doublets or triplets of spikes are recorded from the soma and basal dendrites, the apical dendrites generate slow depolarization waves of different amplitudes, which last as long as the spike burst at the neuron output. The aperiodical changes of the membrane potential in the two asymmetrical apical dendrites are asynchronous during this complex pattern: there is a big difference between the corresponding voltage traces at all stages of the activity.

A high-frequency regular pattern (activation intensity of $15\,\mu S\,cm^{-2}$) in the soma and basal dendrites is formed by repeating doublets of spikes (Figure 13.8, C). Simultaneously recorded activity in the apical dendrites is a synchronously repeating sequence composed of a pair of slow waves of depolarization, which have different amplitudes and are phase-shifted. Hence, during generation of a simple periodical pattern, the membrane potential synchronously oscillates in different parts of the dendritic arborization with a certain shape-dependent phase shift. This indicates synchronous periodical transitions of the whole arborization between the states of low and high depolarization during generation of the simple pattern in the form of a one-event (a doublet) repeating sequence.

This is in contrast to the generation of a quasi-stochastic, aperiodical pattern when asymmetrical parts of the apical dendritic subtree change their states of low and high depolarization asynchronously and their levels of membrane depolarization are noticeably different.

13.4 Some general rules

Interesting rules emerge from the comparison made on the active Purkinje and pyramidal neuron models.

Simple regular auto-rhythmical patterns are generated at low- and high-conductance states and whatever the metrical asymmetry is, all the domains of the dendritic arborizations change their states of low and high depolarization synchronously. At that stage, the difference of potentials (lateral voltage) between different domains is small, presuming small lateral currents and correspondingly, small perturbations of the local current–voltage relations at different dendritic sites. Therefore, the *spatial dendritic signature* of the simple patterns is a spatially homogeneous electrical state of different dendritic domains. Simple patterns mean a meagre repertoire of possible electrical activities in the low- and high-conductance states.

The repertoire of output patterns becomes rich in the medium-conductance range. The patterns become complex, forming a repeating sequence of many elementary events of different types. A relatively small conductance change produces a change in the pattern type, i.e. change in the repeating sequence in terms of the number of elementary events and the duration of the sequence. When a complex multi-event sequence is generated, the asymmetrical parts of the dendritic arborization change their states of low and high membrane potentials asynchronously. During this activity, the lateral voltages between asymmetrical parts of the arborization are large. This is the condition for big lateral currents and, correspondingly, large perturbations of the local current–voltage relations. Therefore, the *spatial dendritic signature* of the diverse complex patterns are made of different combinations of the upstate and downstate depolarizations in discrete dendritic domains of more or less expressed metrical asymmetry.

Specific limits of the synaptic conductance ranges providing poor and rich repertoires depend on the size of the dendritic arborization in different types of neurons (cf. Purkinje and pyramidal neurons) or the size of different parts of the same arborization of a given neuron (cf. apical and basal dendrites of a pyramidal neuron arborization). This size-dependence of the conductance range limits can be roughly estimated by divergence of the passive transfer profiles along asymmetrical subtrees computed at different values of the membrane conductivity G_m (resistivity $R_m = 1/G_m$) (Figure 11.5).

The demonstration that dendritic arborizations with different morphologies and ion channels that display similar variations of repertoires of the output discharge patterns authorizes one to consider this finding to be a general rule for any operating neuron.

References

De Schutter, E. and Bower, J. M. (1994). An active membrane model of the cerebellar Purkinje cell. I. Simulation of current-clamps in slice. *J. Neurophysiol.*, **71**:375–400.

Gutfreund, Y., Yarom, Y. and Segev, I. (1995). Subthreshold oscillations and resonant frequency in guinea-pig cortical neurons: physiology and modelling. *J. Physiol.*, **483**:621–640.

Hamill, O. P., Huguenard, J. R. and Prince, D. A. (1991). Patch-clamp studies of voltage-gated currents in identified neurons of the rat cerebral cortex. *Cereb. Cortex*, 1:48–61.

Korogod, S. M., Kopysova, I. L., Bras, H., Gogan, P. and Tyč-Dumont, S. (1996). Differential back-invasion of a single complex dendrite of an abducens motoneuron by N-methyl-D-aspartate-induced oscillations: a simulation study. *Neuroscience*, **75**:1153–1163.

Kulagina, I. B., Korogod, S. M., Horcholle-Bossavit, G., Batini, C. and Tyč-Dumont, S. (2007). The electrodynamics of the dendritic space in Purkinje cells of the cerebellum. *Arch. Ital. Biol.*, **145**:211–233.

Mainen, Z. F., Joerges, J., Huguenard, J. R. and Sejnowski, T. J. (1995). A model of spike initiation in neocortical pyramidal neurons. *Neuron*, **15**:1427–1439.

Mainen, Z. F. and Sejnowski, T. J. (1996). Influence of dendritic structure on firing pattern in model neocortical neurons. *Nature*, **382**:363–366.

Miyasho, T., Takagi, H., Suzuki, H., Watanabe, M., Inoue, S., Kudo, Y. and Miyakawa, H. (2001). Low-threshold potassium channels and a low-threshold calcium channel regulate Ca^{2+} spike firing in the dendrites of cerebellar Purkinje neurons: a modeling study. *Brain Res.*, **891**:106–115.

Reuveni, I., Friedman, A., Amitai, Y. and Gutnick, M. J. (1993). Stepwise repolarization from Ca^{2+} plateaus in neocortical pyramidal cells: evidence for nonhomogeneous distribution of HVA Ca^{2+} channels in dendrites. *J. Neurosci.*, **13**:4609–4621.

14

Concluding remarks

Coming back from our journey into dendritic space, we bring back with us the conviction that we have discovered some new critical notions which are the messages that we must pass on.

What did we learn about the features pictured in many handbooks under such key words as branching dendrites, complex trees, tapering branches, branching point, excitable dendrites, etc. These words give a feeling of *déjà vu*. Do they really take on a special new significance in the description of operating neuronal dendrites as dynamical electrical devices? We strongly believe that the answer is yes indeed, as we attribute a specific role to every one of these structural features in a harmonious working ensemble!

The scope of our book is restricted to *the dynamical electrical picture of dendritic space*. This picture is composed of spatial profiles of electrical values along dendritic branches. We refer to what is observed as electrical states of parts of the whole dendritic arborization. Mapping these values on the reconstructed images of the dendrites provides a specific mosaic of electrical states of its parts, characterizing the electrical state of the whole arborization. The dendritic structure is both the bearer and determinant of its electrical properties as a whole.

To make these geometric features and the mechanisms underlying their function clearer, we select special artificial conditions which help to unveil some hidden neuronal operations. We use models imperfect and simplified, but efficient to analyze reality. They replace impossible observations by simulations.

In our models, we use the following simplifications:

(1) The specific membrane properties are spatially homogeneous over the whole arborization: everywhere in the dendrites the same cocktail of ion channels is present with the same surface density. Our reason for these simplifications is that we perceive the electrical states of the whole arborization as a mosaic of electrical states of the branches and subtrees. The non-trivial state is when different parts differ in their states

with characteristic electrical values spatially heterogeneous. Since both the membrane properties and inputs are spatially homogeneous, the observed heterogeneity of electrical states of the dendritic sites can only be attributed to the heterogeneity of dendritic geometry due to variation of the branch lengths and diameters, that is the *metrical asymmetry*.

(2) The synaptic activation attributed to the dendrites is exclusively excitatory, homogeneous in space and constant in time. This configuration is qualified in our book as a spatially homogeneous tonic activation of the excitatory membrane conductance.

(3) The electrical maps are considered mainly in the steady state. The steady state means that a given electrical state lasts infinitely, as if the time is frozen. This is 'long enough' to catch the spatial picture of the electrical states and understand the electrical communication between the dendritic sites. By observing the path profiles of the membrane voltage, we see in which directions the voltage drops and hence from where and to where the currents flow over the dendrites. The physical mechanisms of these communications are basic: in a conductive media, the currents flow between sites having different voltages (i.e. electrical states) and this difference is modulated by geometry.

In this context we can summarize our observations and indicate specific and common roles of different structural characteristics of the dendritic arborizations, acting as a whole during the generation of electrical activity of a neuron.

Due to its *branching structure* the dendritic arborization operates as a system of electrically coupled *discrete* elements (branches, subtrees). The coupling takes place at a *branching point*, which is a piece of space much smaller than the whole space of any contacting branch. Such a type of electrical coupling is fundamentally different from that between elements contacting through a wide interface, e.g. like cardiomyocytes forming the continuous excitable media of the myocardium. Such a digitization, splitting into discrete elements, forms the basis for individualization of electrical behaviour of each branch or subtree: the electrical states of sites along a given discrete branch can differ from those along another. This is due to the difference in coupling between internal sites within each branch and between the sites of different branches adjacent to the common branching point.

The *size* of the dendritic arborizations is defined by the the size of its constructive elements: by the lengths and diameters of the branches. The *metrical asymmetry* of branching due to difference in size of the branches is responsible for the difference in electrical load which the coupled branches provide to each other at the branching point. It is this difference in mutual electrical load that makes the basis for difference in electrical states between the coupled discrete elements of the branching dendritic tree. This difference can be smaller or greater, but it always exists between asymmetrical branches and subtrees. However, one cannot justifiably state that this difference is significant or insignificant without having a clear measure of the significance. At this stage of our knowledge of dendritic functioning, we don't have such a measure. It is a new horizon opened up in front of us and we can only assume that derivation of a formal measure of significance of electrical difference between asymmetrical paths may come from further scrutinizing the geometry-induced features of the discharge patterns.

The *complexity* of a system is defined by the number of its discrete elements. In this sense, the dendritic arborization is complex, as it is composed of many branches and subtrees. They can be in similar or dissimilar states i.e. differ insignificantly or significantly. As the electrical state of the whole arborization is determined by a combination of states of the constitutive elements, the *complexity and asymmetry* determine together the number of combinations of states of the elements, and ultimately the diversity of states of the whole arborization. This could be a basis for the formation of more or less rich repertoires of electrical activity patterns generated by the whole neuron in which the dendritic arborization is the largest part, not only as the receiver of the inputs, but also as the generator of the output signal.

14.1 Impact for interpretation of neuronal discharges

During our journey in dendritic space, we have dropped for a while the education in electrophysiology that we have received and that we have taught our students. First of all, this concerns the aspects which are based mainly on the data available with the conventional tools of electrophysiologists, the microelectrode recordings from a single point in the soma or, in better cases, from a few more points located mainly in proximal dendrites. According to the dogma, the dendritic synapse acts and generates local postsynaptic potentials which are transferred to the trigger zone, at the initial segment. The voltage at the trigger zone does or doesn't reach threshold and the neuron does or doesn't fire the action potential. Electrophysiology deals with transient temporal events which are described thoroughly and well analyzed, but fail to explain how a neuron generates the variety of its output discharge patterns.

Now with reference to our preceding accomplishments, old and new concepts must be put together for providing a comprehensive vision of how time and space aspects are united in the whole picture of the output discharge patterns of the neuron. In the dynamic case, the states of different dendritic sites change and the rates of change are different due to the voltage-dependence of kinetic properties of many dendritic channels. When one makes snapshots of electrical states at different moments in time, that is freezing time, the electrical mosaic evolves from one snapshot to another, but the governing rules of electrical communications based on geometry remain the same as in the steady state. We believe that, if the observer's eye is trained to see the geometry-induced features in the spatial electrical maps obtained in conditions of spatially homogeneous properties and in steady states, this may help a lot in finding the corresponding features in more complex natural conditions.

14.2 The dancing dendrites

Chapter 13 provides tools for training the observer to look at the time course of the membrane potential of active dendritic branches during generation of output discharges. This is a striking experience for an electrophysiologist. From now on, each time he records action potentials, he will inevitably imagine the electrical behaviour of the dendrites that are responsible for the temporal events that he knows so well.

Our videos present animation of some examples of the temporal evolution of the dendritic patterns of the transmembrane voltages generated by the neuron during a single cycle of membrane oscillatory activity. The electrical path profiles along each branch move about in a fascinating ballet, orchestrated by their different structural characteristics, acting as a whole during the generation of electrical activity of a neuron. NeuronViewer, developed by Valery Kukushka, is an interactive tool accompanying our book to play the score of the dendritic music that generates the output discharge patterns of the neuron. This imaging device helps to grasp the dendritic signature of the neuronal activity (available at URL www.cambridge.org/9780521896771). Our work reports some of the mechanisms that explain the dendritic origin of the variety of patterns of the output discharges.

14.3 Speculation for the future

The memories brought from our travel to dendritic space require revisiting major aspects of conventional concepts of the neuronal functions and may be thought-provoking for neuroscientists working in different fields. We can share some of our speculations concerning further development of biophysics and physiology of neurons.

14.3.1 The sensitivity function

Particularly, one can speculate about *biophysical mechanisms* by which the electrical dynamics of the complex asymmetrical branching structure of the dendrites govern the repertoire of discharge patterns in different neurons, depending on the intensity of their inputs. One candidate mechanism could be space-dependent sensitivity of the dendritic transfer properties to variation of the membrane conductance, which may change as a result of both activities induced by synaptic action from other neurons and generated intrinsically (Korogod *et al.*, 2000; Kulagina *et al.*,

2007). This aspect requires a systematic study. A similar problem is considered in the theory of control systems of different natures. The so-called sensitivity functions are used as a standard complementary to the transfer functions of a system and this tool might help in providing exhaustive descriptions of the transfer properties of the neuronal dendrites. Differential parameter sensitivities of the transfer properties of asymmetrical dendritic paths could be a pre-requisite for dynamic geometry-dependent reconfiguration of the electrical structure of the dendritic arborizations. In this context, it is also worthwhile to study how the sensitivity depends on the range of variation of electrical parameters. As we have demonstrated in this book (Chapters 11–13) the mosaic of electrical states of asymmetrical parts of the dendritic arborization is most diverse when the values of the dendritic membrane conductance are in some intermediate range, which is related to the size of the arborization. This situation can be termed the 'mid-conductance state' by analogy with the widely used term 'high-conductance state'. Detailed consideration of electrical communication between asymmetrical domains of the arborization in the mid-conductance state can open new perspectives for understanding the structural pre-requisites for the diversity of discharge patterns of morphologically complex neurons.

14.3.2 The functional dendritic space

The fixed shapes of dendritic arborizations drawn by anatomists since Ramón y Cajal can be revisited in terms of the dynamic functionality of the neuron. If we accept that the artificial conditions of our simulation mimic different states of neuronal activity and that neurons are spontaneously active in their networks, the synaptic background activity must have an impact on the size and shape of the functional dendritic field.

The spatial reconfiguration of charge transfer effectiveness in active dendritic arborization opens the question of the pre- and postsynaptic scenarios when the neuron is bombarded by the synaptic systems. The great majority of the studies focus upon the synaptic connections. The presynaptic factors, as well as the postsynaptic membrane receptors are extensively analyzed. Meanwhile the role of the electrical states of the dendritic membrane per se as the receiving target is rarely addressed. We suggest that the synaptic afferent systems to single neurons meet different domains of the dendritic membrane which display different transfer efficiencies at a given time. For example, our results obtained in Purkinje neurons show spatial dendritic sectors separated by a difference in voltage as high as about 100 mV during a single membrane oscillation (see Chapter 13). As a consequence, these functional dendritic sectors, which are alternatively turned on and off during a cycle, may be a plastic device for selecting synaptic inputs.

14.3.3 Invitation for other journeys in dendritic space

Our book is an attempt to extract some specific structural features that can explain how a neuron implements the variety of its output discharges patterns. Our wish is to provide a toolkit for understanding the biophysical mechanisms that explain the processing and for predicting how different shapes of dendritic arborizations will generate different output patterns.

Despite the progress made in the last decades, much is in front of us. The combination of different approaches will bring new complexities and new variability that characterize various levels, together with new results. The experimental verification of our spatial hypothesis requires complementing the conventional approaches with new tools that provide a full description of the local transmembrane potential in the dendritic membrane over large regions of the arborization. Cellular imaging with voltage-sensitive dyes acting as a sensor of the local electrical field in the neuronal membrane have already furnished some results (Gogan *et al.*, 1995; Zecevic, 1996; Savtchenko *et al.*, 2001; Djurisic *et al.*, 2004; Milojkovic *et al.*, 2005) and are progressing with better dyes and better optics. Biotechnology will produce molecular machines that will manipulate the microstructure of the neuronal membrane by drug delivery systems with controlled release (Browne and Feringa, 2006; Hutzler *et al.*, 2006; Lichtenberger and Fromherz, 2007). Fabrication of controlled dendritic morphologies on micro-arrays (Katz and Grinvald, 2002; Jimbo, 2007) are no longer in the domain of imagination. The interpretation of the results obtained with each new approach is often puzzling and will require new hypotheses from new efforts in mathematics, biophysics, engineering and neurobiology.

References

Browne, W. R. and Feringa, B. L. (2006). Making molecular machines work. *Nature Nanotechnology*, **1**:25–35.

Djurisic, M., Antic, S., Chen, W. R. and Zecevic, D. (2004). Voltage imaging from dendrites of mitral cells: EPSP attenuation and spike trigger zones. *J. Neurosci.*, **24**:6703–6714.

Gogan, P., Schmidel-Jakob, I., Chitti, Y. and Tyč-Dumont, S. (1995). Fluorescence imaging of local membrane electric fields during the excitation of single neurons in culture. *Biophys. J.*, **69**:299–310.

Hutzler, M., Lambacher, A., Eversmann, B., Jenkner, M., Thewes, R. and Fromherz, P. (2006). High-resolution multi-transistor array recording of electrical field potentials in cultured brain slices. *J. Neurophysiol.*, **96**:1638–1645.

Jimbo, Y. (2007). MEA-based recording of neuronal activity in vitro. *Arch. Ital. Biol.*, **145**:289–297.

Katz, L. C. and Grinvald, A. (2002). New technologies: molecular probes, microarrays, microelectrodes, microscopes and MRI. *Curr. Opin. Neurobiol.*, **12**:551–553.

Korogod, S. M., Kulagina, I. B., Horcholle-Bossavit, G., Gogan, P. and Tyč-Dumont, S. (2000). Activity-dependent reconfiguration of the effective dendritic field of motoneurons. *J. Comp. Neurol.*, **422**:18–34.

Kulagina, I. B., Korogod, S. M., Horcholle-Bossavit, G., Batini, C. and Tyč-Dumont, S. (2007). The electrodynamics of the dendritic space in Purkinje cells of the cerebellum. *Arch. Ital. Biol.*, **145**:211–233.

Lichtenberger, J. and Fromherz, P. (2007). A cell-semiconductor synapse: transistor recording of vesicle release in chromaffin cells. *Biophys. J.*, **92**:2262–2268.

Milojkovic, B. A., Radojicic, M. S. and Antic, S. D. (2005). A strict correlation between dendritic and somatic plateau potential depolarizations in the rat prefontal cortex pyramidal neurons. *J. Neurosci.*, **25**:3940–3951.

Savtchenko, L., Gogan, P., Korogod, S. M. and Tyč-Dumont, S. (2001). Imaging stochastic spatial variability of active channel clusters during excitation of single neurons. *Neurosci. Res.*, **39**:431–446.

Zecevic, D. (1996). Multiple spike-initiation zones in single neurons revealed by voltage-sensitive dyes. *Nature*, **381**:322–325.

Index

Printed in the United States
by Baker & Taylor Publisher Services